SENIORCISE

*A Simple Guide
to Fitness for the
Elderly and Disabled*

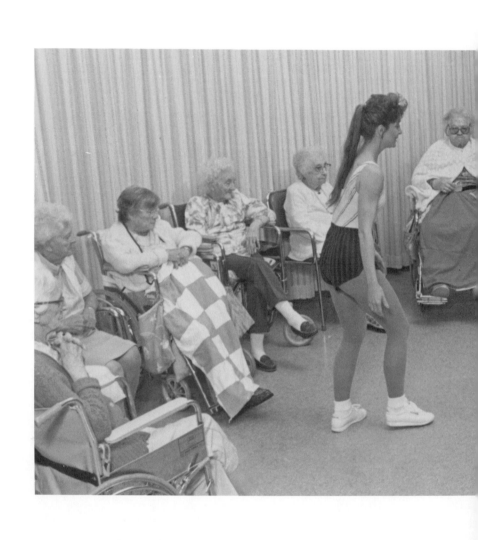

SENIORCISE

A Simple Guide to Fitness for the Elderly and Disabled

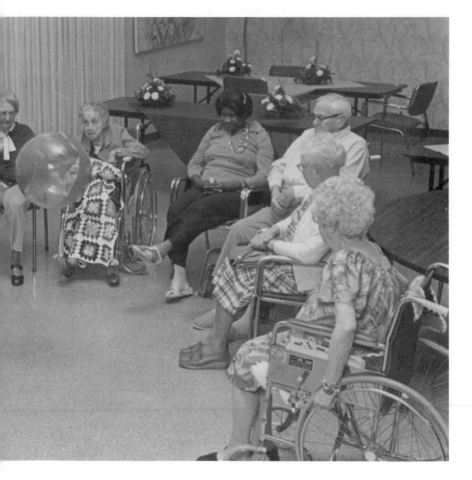

JANIE CLARK

Pineapple Press • Sarasota, FL

Inquiries should be addressed to Pineapple Press, Inc., P.O. Drawer 16008, Sarasota, Florida 34239.

Library of Congress Cataloging-in-Publication Data

Clark, Janie, 1956-
    Seniorcise : a simple guide to fitness for the elderly and disabled
/ by Janie Clark. — 1st ed.
    p.   cm.
    ISBN 0-910923-55-8 : $14.95
    1. Aged—Health and hygiene.   2. Exercise for the aged.   3. Aged,
Physically handicapped—Health and hygiene.   I. Title.
    RA777.6.C57 1988
613'.0438—dc19   88-25062
                                                                        CIP

1st Edition
    10 9 8 7 6 5 4 3 2 1

Design by Joan Lange Kresek
Composition by Lubin Typesetting, Inc., Sarasota, Florida
Printed and bound by BookCrafters, Fredericksburg, Virginia

TO MY PARENTS

ACKNOWLEDGMENTS

The author wishes to thank the many professionals whose experience and knowledge contributed toward the development of the Seniorcise program: researchers, doctors, nurses, physical therapists, exercise specialists, and recreators. Special thanks go to the residents of Ocean View Nursing Home in New Smyrna Beach, Florida, and to their families as well as to the nursing home staff for all their help in the making of this book. The photo art in *Seniorcise* is by Debbie Norman and Steighner Studio of New Smyrna Beach, Florida, and the author's hair/makeup is by Daytona Beach Community College Cosmetology School under Director Michael Kirk.

TABLE OF CONTENTS

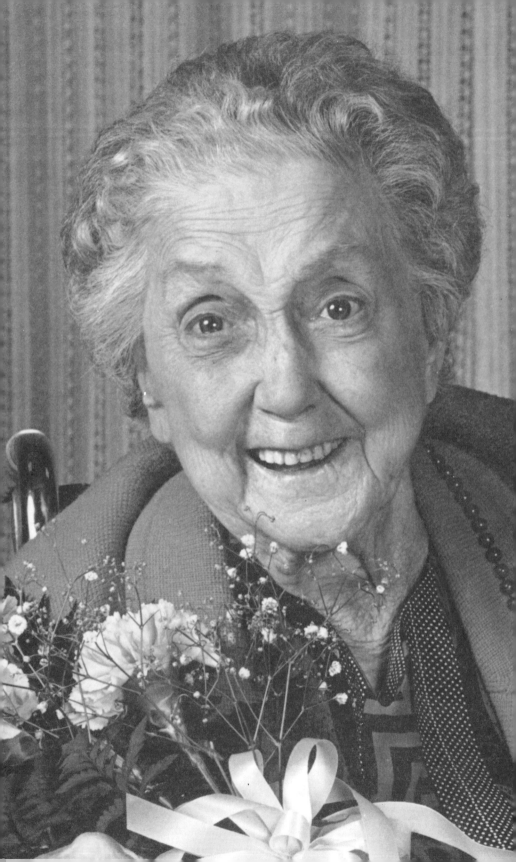

INTRODUCTION

What has come over quiet little Ocean View Nursing Home? That's what townspeople in New Smyrna Beach, Florida, wondered when the newspaper showed a ragtag troupe of preteen breakdancers windmilling and moonwalking before an audience of swaying, clapping retirees.

The answer is, simply, a fun approach to geriatric fitness.

SENIORCISE: The Program

The elderly segment of our American population is burgeoning. In fact, the U.S. Bureau of the Census found that 2,796,000 Americans were eighty-five years old or older in 1986. By the year 2000, the count is expected to approach five million. By 2020, it will exceed seven million.

And yet, concerning physical exercise, this group continues to be neglected.

This book will provide complete directions for implementing my three-part fitness program for very elderly and disabled senior citizens. The key components of the program are: 1) calisthenic exercise, 2) sit-down sports, and 3) intellectually stimulating games designed to discourage mental backsliding.

Supplemental ideas will be given for special activities that range from icebreaker games to dance demonstrations like the one described above.

Pointers on how to manage elderly fitness classes will be discussed in detail.

A separate chapter about one-on-one fitness supervision should prove helpful to those working with solitary persons and special cases. And, a final chapter on parting company will list useful steps a fitness leader can take when students return to the care of their families or transfer to other nursing homes.

All the instructions will emphasize the important roles of warmth and gladness in conducting a well-balanced fitness plan for the very elderly.

How It Came About

As an experienced fitness professional, I have supervised many exercise programs and have enjoyed working with children, young adults, middle-aged persons, and senior citizens. So, on a professional level, I was both intrigued and excited upon receiving the offer to administer a nursing home fitness program.

On a more personal level, I was equally pleased.

I grew up in one of South Carolina's tiny, close-knit farming communities where many a morning was spent calling on "shut-in" neighbors with my mother. Hometown church groups also sought to serve the aged and, through them, I often visited nursing homes in nearby towns.

During these early experiences, I learned to love and admire our seniorest senior citizens. Later, I hoped for a chance to contribute to their well-being through my work.

Solving the Problems

After signing the necessary contracts, I set about to plan the new program. Very quickly, I discovered a shortage of useable information on meeting the needs of my new exercise students.

There was plenty of literature on recreation and exercise for the *active* over-65 set. But most of the works I was able to locate relating to programs for the physically restricted seemed long, technical, and void of good illustrations depicting exercises appropriate for my students.

Some very fine books included chapter after chapter on arts, crafts, party ideas, and other activities irrelevant to planning a program for fitness.

I noticed that in some books the instructions for many games began with the words: *Pass out pencil and paper.* But most of my students either couldn't hold pencils or couldn't see well enough to enjoy writing-games.

Many discussion activities required participants to research the topics in advance. This was clearly more than I could ask of my new fitness students.

Exercise recommendations included running in place and swimming. But my group were mostly wheelchair-restricted. Many of the students were stroke victims with severely limited movement. And, besides, there was no swimming pool!

I knew I needed a brand-new fitness plan, one that would be just right for my special nursing home students. Now, thanks to their patience and help, I do have a program that works for them. And, in the following pages, I'd like to share its basic principles with you.

Who This Book Is For

This book is for severely restricted and semi-restricted elderly persons and for all the people who seek to work productively with them.

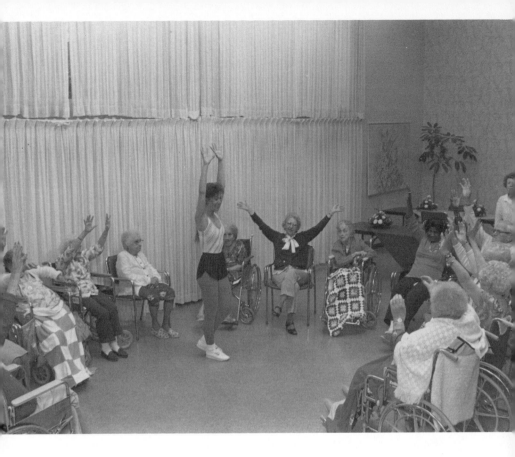

If you have a loved one residing in a retirement home, does his home provide him with an adequate program of exercise and physical recreation? This book can help you to answer that question. Compare the fitness activities offered at his nursing home with those of the program described in this book. Does his home's fitness agenda include all of the components needed for a well-balanced fitness program? If not, you (or someone else authorized by the facility) can use this book to start one.

This book is also meant to assist exercise professionals, social workers, nursing home activities coordinators, and other geriatric employees. In listening to nursing home activities coordinators, I have noticed one major recurrent theme. Many wish to expand their fitness programs, but they have so many other responsibilities that there is no time left to personally supervise any new, regularly scheduled activities. At the same time, training an assistant to run a responsible geriatric fitness program — encompassing specific exercises, cognitive and sensory games, sports adaptations, safety precautions, medical considerations, management principles, motivational techniques, and so much more — is nearly as time-prohibitive as doing it oneself! This book, then, can be used as a text in the training of activities assistants. I hope that it will also prove useful as a training tool for other recreation personnel and as an aid to continuing-education managers who are responsible for providing certified service leaders to their communities.

One main purpose of this book is to offer fitness guidance to family members caring for convalescent or infirm loved ones at home. For clarity's sake, the book is addressed to group leaders in retirement centers, but most of the tips and instructions can easily be adapted to private use by responsible relatives. Chapter Seven, "Working with the Elderly One-on-One," will be of special interest to families.

Another group that I particularly hope to reach with this book includes the many fine volunteers who serve society's oldest. Every day sincere individuals and civic organizations donate long hours to grateful nursing home facilities. The problem is that workaday staff members don't always have time to indoctrinate volunteers. As a result, they all too often wind up handing out cupcakes or leading childish games to pass the time. I hope this book will help to supply effective channels for the talents and energies of these invaluable people.

Many of the following activities can also be employed in fitness programs for non-elderly participants. Active seniors at community centers, congregate living complexes, and private boarding homes will benefit from the recreational exercises. Temporarily or permanently disabled persons of *all* ages will appreciate having a selection of seated activities they can perform. And children, especially, will thoroughly enjoy testing their creative abilities with the games.

To the Point

Since I do want the book to be useful to both lay and paid workers, I have made an effort to keep descriptions and explanations simple. In other words, if you are a non-professional (or if you are new to the business) you don't need any formal training or any specific educational background to be able to utilize the program. If you are an experienced professional, I hope that you will discover some fresh ideas to incorporate into your ongoing work.

Whether you are a paid professional, a volunteer, or a concerned family member — the fact that you are involved in geriatric care implies that you don't have time for a long, ponderous volume full of scholarly theories. I know that when starting our new fitness program, what I needed was a practical handbook with straightforward guidelines for effective interaction with the elderly and with clear-cut directions for beneficial fitness activities that I could lead. The last thing I needed was a list of activities that required long preparation time or costly props and materials.

For these reasons, this book is pared down to a concise treatment. When nursing home residents are described, their names have been changed to protect their privacy. Elderly exercise participants will be called "students" or "members," just as people of other age groups are called when they participate in exercise classes. You will be called the "leader." For every how-to direction in the following text, the preparation is already completed. Each activity has already been tested on my students, then modified, if necessary, to get the "bugs" out. In fact, this work is comprised of favorites of my elderly fitness students.

Instead of illustrating the principles of this program with dry statistics and figures, I have used real examples of my students' experiences. After all, you're not working with charts and graphs and numerical data. You're working with real, feeling, hoping human beings who are counting on you to enrich their latter years.

The Rewards

And this train of thought leads us to an agreeable fact about geriatric fitness supervision. The students on the receiving end of what you have to offer also have something to offer you: the joy and satisfaction of seeing your work count for others *and* all the wisdom and love they have stored over the many years.

My group alone has included a daring female sea captain, a tough veteran of Kentucky's dangerous coal mines, and one lady who made a living performing in her husband's dance band — proud people who have taken risks and lived many exciting years. They may require help to get along now, but their independent spirits are still very much in evidence. And they are waiting, ready to welcome the person who will recognize, respect, and encourage that special individuality.

I hope this book will help you to be that person.

God bless you,
Janie Clark

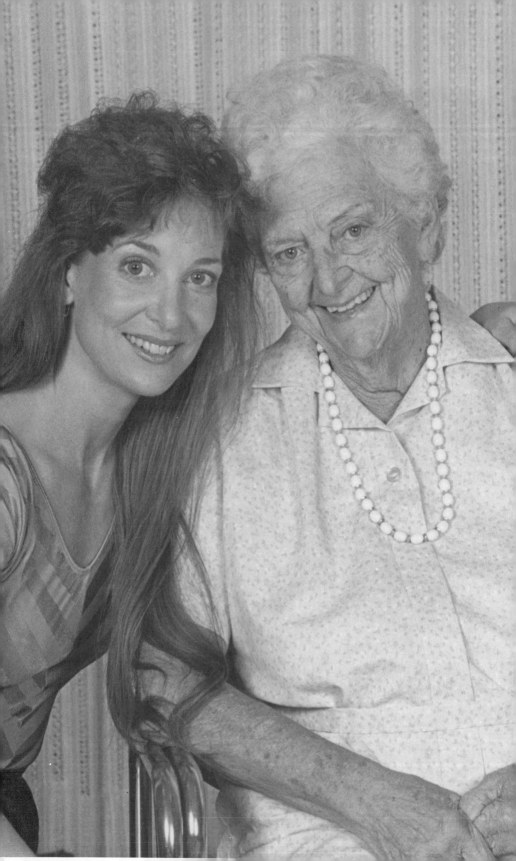

CHAPTER 1

Supervising a Class of Elderly Students: Do's and Don't's

Here's Your Challenge

As a geriatric fitness leader, you are expected to walk into a room full of elderly strangers — each of whom is to some extent disabled by conditions that range from tumors and stroke to Alzheimer's and heart disease — and earn their confidence and cooperation in order to lead them in a worthwhile fitness program.

Now before you accept this challenge, consider the fact that some of your students may exceed one hundred years of age and that your class is likely to include both male and female members. One may be deaf and another blind. One singsongs an enigmatic chant. Another's eyes are bright and alert, but he is unable to speak. Some are missing fingers — some, legs and feet. Several can move only the limbs on one side of their bodies. One is asleep, clutching a well-worn Raggedy Ann doll. Almost everyone is confined to a wheelchair. Several are settled in comfortably, observing you pleasantly with polite expectation.

Are you ready to deal with this fitness group effectively? Being ready with viable lesson plans is half the job, and this book will help you with that preparation. But of equal importance in this type of work is the way in which you respond to your aged students. The way you act will largely determine how they, in turn, react to you.

A geriatric fitness leader needs to be a singular sort of professional, one who desires to enhance life for the elderly and who, at the same time, wants a challenging occupation in which creativity and imagination really count.

In this field, your personal attitude towards the elderly will be extremely significant. Remember that acting standoffish or even a little frightened around the aged won't help to accomplish your goals or theirs. But showing that you care in an artless, natural manner creates a setting in which students and leader are able to learn and progress together.

Building Trust

If your initial group classes fail to set the world on fire, don't be too discouraged. It takes time to win the trust and loyalty necessary for lively fitness meetings.

Nursing home residents have encountered well-meaning guests who unknowingly condescended to them. They have had visitors who suggested fatuous pastimes or who just couldn't think of anything to say. They have known plenty of people who came to their home a few times, only to disappear with no explanation. For all they know, you may be one of these people, too. You will have to demonstrate otherwise.

Your Voice: "Would You Mind Speaking Up a Little?"

For starters, don't talk baby talk to grown-ups! Do speak distinctly and at a moderate rate of speed.

Keep in mind that just because someone is older, it does not automatically follow that he is hard-of-hearing. Now how would you like it if someone persistently shouted in your ear for no good reason? Nursing home residents are not a homogeneous group with fixed traits. Each individual is unique, and it is your job to respect that. Just ask nursing home employees to identify students with hearing disabilities. Then you can set a volume level that best suits the needs of your group. Consider having students with marked hearing loss sit directly beside you during fitness class. Or, when giving instructions, walk over and stand next to a student who you know is hard-of-hearing.

By watching for students' faces to register signs of comprehension, you can determine when you need to repeat yourself. A good rule of thumb (especially when starting a new class) is to state all specific directions twice. Seat students in a circle; this will enable them to see and hear both you and each other better. Deliver instructions first towards the students on one side of the circle, then paraphrase the instructions while facing the other side of the circle.

Peripheral sounds and commotions that you find easy to tune out may, nevertheless, prove distracting and unnerving to your students. At the beginning of class, you may need to close doors that allow noise in from residence hallways or employee break rooms. If your group meets in a cafeteria, be sure to minimize kitchen clatter by closing the doors between work areas and the dining hall.

Wheelchair Etiquette

Leaning on someone's wheelchair is a thoughtless act that he may consider tantamount to leaning against his person.

In close conversation with a wheelchair user, kneel on the floor or sit down

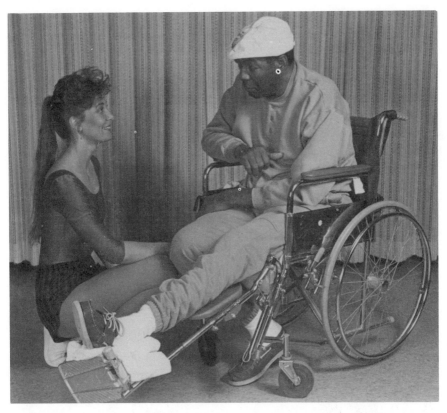

across from him. Do not compel him to crane his neck looking up at you.

Offering to push a student's wheelchair when you're headed his way is considerate. Pushing away without asking first is presumptuous.

Reach Out and Touch

The value of physically touching your students just cannot be stressed too much. Many nursing home residents do not receive regular visitors. Their primary physical contact with other human beings may be limited to events such as being helped from bed to wheelchair and other day-to-day care procedures. Most will welcome a hearty pat on the shoulder (just not on the head, please) and other brotherly tokens of physical affection. In fact, it may be difficult for us to understand just how much a friendly touch might mean to a given student in fitness class.

Touching can be a good icebreaker, particularly for a brand new group. Try walking around your group circle while shaking hands and speaking personally to everyone in attendance. To make the class even more cohesive, have everyone turn and shake hands with his neighbor on either side. This simple activity has brought so many smiles to so many of my students that I have sometimes gone around the circle three or four times shaking hands. (See Chapter Four for more icebreakers.)

Also, remember the power of touch for reinforcing active participation habits. When you notice that a particular student is working very hard, you might just casually wander over and drape your arm around his neck. At the same time, verbally compliment the fine job that he is doing. That small bit of recognition might just be the impetus that brings this student back to your next fitness meeting.

The same principle holds true when you observe that a student's attention is straying. From his point of view, a good-natured tickle is not such a bad way to get nudged back into action.

On the other hand, do be sensitive to the fact that a student may prefer not to be touched. Although this is a rare characteristic, it is one you should remember in order to respect the rights of your students.

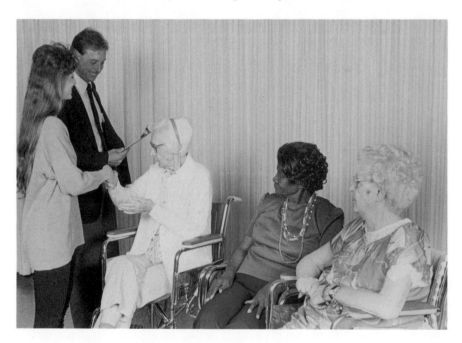

Getting Personal with Your Students

How much more effective do you think the icebreaker, handshaking, would be if you called each student by his name as you took his hand and greeted him? Plenty more effective! So do make the effort to learn students' names fast. You can speed up this process by giving each member a name tag to wear during the first few meetings. Some students will lose their tags between meetings, so either remember to collect them at the end of class or to carry an adequate supply of fresh ones. During subsequent meetings, use their names every time you get a chance. Let them know you appreciate them as distinguished individuals.

And, speaking of individuals, learn about their limitations — yes, even if it means sitting through a complaint session on ailments and operations. The information that Mary Jones has no mobility in her left leg is vital to the supervision of her fitness program. You will want to make certain that her wheelchair is angled so that the other foot is prominent during kickball games.

Likewise, pay attention to students' strong points as well as to which events different students enjoy the most. Mary Jones has a bad left leg but she may, however, own a terrific pitching arm. Participating in the "wastebasket toss" might improve her eye-hand coordination, and thus significantly enhance her ability to carry out daily tasks.

Focusing in this way on a student's strengths (while working to decrease his limitations) will help him to build and fortify a positive self-image. Imagine the impact of a confidence booster like this on someone who may have been feeling blue about being cared for in a hospital setting.

Letting Students Get Personal with You

If you arrive like clockwork for each class, if you come prepared with planned activities, if you touch your students and learn their names, and yet fail to reveal a little of yourself — then you will never engage your group's attention to the degree that inspires optimal fitness performance. In effect, you will be just another professional who comes in and dispenses a service. You won't be one of them.

So loosen up! You don't have to tell these folks about any skeletons in your closet. But you might share some details about your hobbies or your pets. Tell them about your garden. Let them in on the news that your family is house-hunting. Describe the high-school reunion you attended over the weekend.

Of course you wouldn't want to bore your students with too many particulars about your personal life. But do let them get to know you as a full-fledged person with human feelings and personal goals. Initially, it will help them to place your face and remember you from one meeting to the next. In the long run, they will appreciate your openness and will respond with more interest in you and in what you have to offer.

Chatting: A Good Old-fashioned Fitness Tool

Informal chatting sets a relaxed atmosphere that inclines elderly students to enjoy taking part in planned activities. By encouraging casual conversation, a little when you arrive and a little all along throughout the meeting, you will demonstrate that your students are as important to you as your scheduled program is. Reluctance to take occasional social breaks could make you seem, at best, like a stuffed shirt and, at worst, like a drill sergeant. If you give that impression, students may not be back for more classes. Keep in mind that their participation is voluntary.

Now I'm not recommending that you allow your fitness meeting to degenerate into a free-for-all fellowship hour. Use your position as the leader to provide direction to conversation. After a time, guide it around to the next game or exercise on your agenda.

The Many Uses of Humor

A humorless geriatric fitness program would be a dire proposition indeed. On the other hand, good times tend to foster good results. And you do want to have fun, don't you? Your elderly students do!

With that in mind, look for opportunities to amuse the members of your class. Sharing a new joke at each meeting is one good policy, and your bookstore can furnish appropriate joke books and magazines. Better yet, try to incorporate humor as a fundamental element of your overall program.

When I talk about the use of humor in a program for the elderly, I'm not referring only to quips, riddles, or stories that build up to funny punch lines. Perhaps *good humor* would be a better expression for the merry mood a leader can set by radiating wit and playfulness himself.

For example, if a resident you pass in the lobby says he's not planning to attend your class, you can't force him to go. You could, however, try a little good humor, like: "Come on, George! You'll make me cry if you skip class today. Have you ever seen a grown woman trying to sob and do leg lifts at the same time?" Or, "How are you going to chase the nurses if you don't exercise to keep up your strength?"

Once class is under way, there are many openings in which to inject good humor. Exercises can be coupled with funny descriptions such as this: "Pretend that the doctor is coming at you with a giant spoonful of horrible-tasting medicine. Now what are you going to do? Close your mouth TIGHT!"

Humor is an excellent instrument with which to chide wayward students. Wearing a friendly expression, use admonishments that will tend to make members feel frisky, like: "Now look what's happened! I turned my back, and this whole side of the room quit exercising. What's that famous saying? While the cat's away, the mice will play. But now I've caught you rats!"

When a student is having an "off" day, he may become sullen, cross, or irate. Try some good-natured teasing to turn his mood around: "Oh, dear! Albert's fussing at me. Now I'm in trouble. Albert, do you know what you are? You're irascible, that's what!" By the time you are finished, the rest of your members will be laughing, and Albert will probably be feeling pretty special and more like himself again.

Convert mistakes into humorous situations. For instance, if Frances kicks the ball wild and sends it outside the field of play, she may be angry at herself for making a bad kick. As you run to retrieve the ball, you can keep her spirits high with a jest, such as: "Here's a lady who really packs a wallop in her kick! Where did that ball get to anyway? Kalamazoo?"

Likewise, if Anna's lap blanket slides, leaving her in an immodest situation, she is likely to feel embarrassed and others may chuckle at her predicament. As you right the blanket, take a positive, light approach by saying: "Anna gets an A-plus for moving enough to rock the boat!" Everyone else can laugh all they want and, now, so can Anna!

These examples have shown some ways that a leader can put humor to work for his students. Keep on the lookout for further opportunities as they present themselves during your meetings. As you can see, adding a touch of levity to your plan can help, not only to make fitness fun, but also to facilitate the smooth operation of your program.

When To Be Firm

Some situations call for stronger medicine than humor. If lighter measures fail to correct a problem, it is sometimes appropriate to take an insistent or firm position. Remember, though, that it is *never* appropriate to be impatient or to get flustered or angry. Below are some typical situations that have occurred in my classes which I have used firmness to resolve.

If a student becomes temporarily disoriented, he may begin to repeat, in a loud voice, some word or phrase that has made a strong impression on his mind. Specific examples that have come up in my group have included the terms *ice cream, green, England,* and *take us home.* In these instances polite requests, touching, and humor all failed to stop the student from chanting. I have had success, however, by combining firmness with diversion. Example: "Betty, hush. Hush now. Lift your arms up. There, that's right." Other members will appreciate your taking the responsibility to end a grating interruption. They will respect you for it, too, if you handle it calmly and courteously.

By the same token, sometimes it is necessary to have a student removed from class. This solution is in order only when the student cannot control his actions and you see that he is disturbing your other members.

In one such case, a student who had attended my class successfully before began to clutch and claw at the other members. In another instance, one uninhibited woman removed all her clothes to the utter dismay of all present. At these times, it is best to summon an aid to take the offender away. But remember that while the student is confused, he may perceive that he is being banished. A cheerful farewell could help to settle his nerves. Then as soon as possible, get the others back to their normal routine. If they criticize or laugh about the other student's behavior, do not try to ignore the event by pretending it didn't happen. Instead, make a truthful comment, like: "Maybe Ella can join us again soon on a better day. I hope so."

I had a tricky situation on my hands one day when one of my best students began shouting at a passerby. It seems that this woman, also a resident of the nursing home, had taken Margaret's newspaper earlier at breakfast. The argument that ensued was rowdy enough to bring our exercise efforts to an abrupt halt. I told Margaret that the middle of fitness class was no place to settle a grievance, but the uproar and indictments continued. Trying to maintain order, I offered to push the women, both of whom were wheelchair-restricted, to another room where they could work out their dispute. I proposed that we call in a qualified staff member to arbitrate.

But they ignored me and the ruckus, in fact, grew louder! Finally I began wheeling Margaret towards the door away from the group.

"I just can't allow this type of disruption," I explained. "It isn't fair to the other students."

Margaret wanted to stay in class more than she wanted to do battle and quickly agreed to settle the spat later. The other lady went on her way, and class proceeded in a normal manner.

Afterwards, I accompanied Margaret to her room, talking things over along the way. She agreed to accept help from the staff member mentioned earlier. I admitted that she'd had "a bone to pick" but added, "I know you can understand that I can't have a sideshow going on at the expense of the others in fitness class." I knew that Margaret was cognizant. She could appreciate a logical reminder that causing a disturbance during class was unacceptable. But, also being a perfectionist, she needed reassurance that I still regarded her as a good student.

In this case, knowing a student's strengths helped in applying the proper action. Margaret is still one of my tiptop members and never misses a meeting.

(I did, by the way, report that matter to the proper staff member, who was instrumental in resolving it. You should report any potential social, mental, or physical problems that you notice among retirement home residents. You will also need to know the location of the nearest alarm signal switch, which you will press only in the event of a medical emergency during class.)

To summarize briefly, be loving, be funny, be cordial and understanding. When intolerable behavior persists, be polite but firm and insistent. Use your authority. Be reasonable. Take the indicated action in a fair and respectful manner.

A Slow, Natural Pace

Since inevitable interruptions and other unknown variables are likely to affect the running of a nursing home fitness class, pacing is one of the keys to a successful program. Keep in mind that some of your students have aches and pains; they might tire easily; their attention spans may not be what they used to be. Too much information delivered too fast or too much nonstop activity could prove overwhelming and unpleasant for them. For these reasons, keep the pace of the class unhurried.

Sometimes class might start a few minutes late since many of the students need assistance getting to and from meetings. You can lend a hand by helping the student who fears he might lose his way or who faces a long wheelchair trip from his room to the meeting room. Be sure to allot a few spare minutes to help out after class as well. Cooperate with the nurses, who may be trying to encourage certain residents to wheel their own vehicles without aid. Also, remember that because of insurance considerations, certain tasks (such as operating Hoyer lifts to raise patients out of bed) can only be performed by certified staff members. When in doubt, ask first.

During class, you may find it necessary to get a glass of water for a coughing student or to help another to the bathroom and back.

Consequently, try not to worry if you don't get to cover all the ground you had planned to during a given meeting. Just save the leftover activities for another day. Don't make your students nervous by racing from one exercise to another. Do pause occasionally to rest or to chat, as we discussed earlier in the chapter. Take the time to introduce each new activity properly, explaining the purpose of the assignment. For example, point to your arm as you say, "This exercise will strengthen your biceps to help you lift objects you want to pick up."

Excuse any member who asks to leave, but make a point to invite him back. Try to see to it that he attends the next meeting that you hold.

Be flexible. If a fitness task reminds a student of an amusing story, make the time to let him share it with your other members. It may spark off some laughter which, after all, is the best medicine. Besides, if you discourage communication now, you will have a hard time drawing it forth on demand later when you are trying to start a group discussion.

Just slow down. Your students are not in a big rush. Don't you be, either.

Planning Your Format

Ideally, fitness class should be held three to four times spaced out over the course of a week to enable the members to achieve lasting benefits. The length of each meeting might reasonably range from one hour to an hour and a half, although that certainly will not consist of continuous physical exercise. Thirty minutes of exercise at one time is enough and even that should be built up to gradually.

Divide the meeting into different periods in order to make it interesting and in order to include all three components of your balanced fitness program: 1) a supervised exercise workout, 2) a special activity or sports event, and 3) an intellectual game designed to promote mental fitness. This adds up to twenty minutes per segment in an hour-long class or thirty minutes per segment in a ninety-minute class.

But don't be a stickler when it comes to timing. Some games take longer than others to play, and you can never predict whether a group discussion will wind down after fifteen minutes or continue with zest for forty-five. Special activities, such as guest performers, may stir up enough excitement to fatigue the members in a briefer than usual length of time. During any particular meeting, you may want to extend an activity that you notice the students are especially enjoying. Remember that a few minutes here and there should be allotted for greeting, resting, and socializing. In other words, even a ninety-minute meeting will never contain enough activity to exhaust the participants. If, infrequently, a meeting is adjourned five or ten minutes before time is up, members will enjoy the change of routine much as they did when classes let out early during their school days. On the other hand, meetings may run into overtime when the students are engrossed in a pleasurable project.

Be alert to the facets of your format that inspire the most participation and to the facets that might be improved. When I began my fitness program, I frequently varied the order of segments within the basic format. I thought that my students would enjoy the variety. But I found that they thrived instead on regularity. They performed best when they knew what was coming next. I got better results by switching to a consistent schedule of exercise first (followed by a short break), kickball or other sports events next, and intellectual games last. Special activities were included occasionally to ward off possible monotony.

Your group may prefer a variable schedule to a fixed one. Or, you may discover that they enjoy kickball so much that they do their best when it is always included in the format to the virtual exclusion of other sports.

Finally, your format should be loose enough to accommodate surprises. For instance, if a Girl Scout troop happens to visit the nursing home during the first part of class, it would be much more fun to let the girls help out with a ball game than it would be to have them sit down and watch calisthenics.

Music: Knowing When It Is a Plus, Knowing When It Is a Minus

Many nursing home residents enjoy working out to music just as much as today's sophisticated spa members do. But you will quickly discover that Mitch Miller and the Lennon Sisters are much preferred to any recording

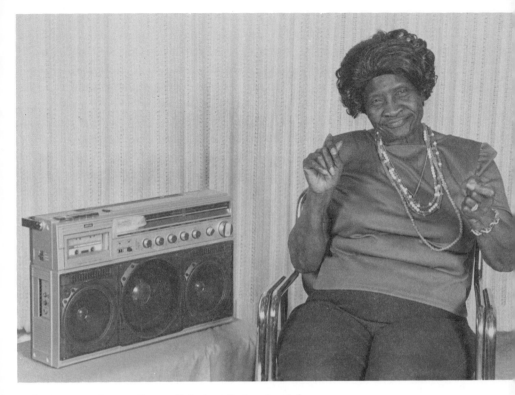

artists currently on the radio's top forty charts!

Fitness groups are made up of individuals, and what works for one group is not necessarily the answer for another. Where music is concerned, be observant. Is the music you are incorporating serving to stimulate members to join in the action? Or, is it taking their attention away from your workouts and sports events?

One duty of the modern spa instructor that you don't have to worry about as a geriatric fitness leader is matching exercise motions exactly to the musical beat (except for choreographed wheelchair dance, which we will discuss in Chapter Four). The nursing home student does not want the volume as loud as a twenty-year-old aerobic dancer does. Music can play softly in the background to enhance the atmosphere and spirit of the class. If movements do go with the beat, then that is a bonus. But remember that trying to ensure that exercises always match the rhythm can put undue pressure on you as well as on your students. It can detract from your flexibility to stop and help individual members or to pause for general explanations.

If you play good musical selections, don't be surprised when some of your students take time-outs for clapping, finger snapping, and singing. This kind of enthusiasm is of value, so if a student occasionally misses a few leg lifts over it — well, it's worth it.

Then again, if students get so carried away by the tunes that they neglect planned activities or spend too much time debating whether the volume is too high or low, you will want to cut back on its use. In that case, consider restricting music to the portion of the class during which concentration is unimportant (such as while you are adjusting individual wheelchairs to make certain that brakes and other features are set right for specific activities).

Once you have determined where and how music fits into your program, there remains the pleasant task of picking out records or tapes. Some of the musical artists that my students like are Benny Goodman, Louis Armstrong, the Andrews Sisters, Billie Holiday, Jim Nabors, and Julie Andrews. Music by any performer who is remembered fondly by your students is a good choice.

Other styles of music that are fun to play at fitness meetings include marches, ballets, symphony overtures, show tunes, ragtime, boogie-woogie, and gospel.

Don't forget that many nursing home residents spend a good deal of time watching television. If they like to keep up with current events, they may enjoy hearing the latest country music hits. The same holds true for light rock 'n' roll. In fact, I asked my group one day if they had ever heard of the rock 'n' roll celebrity, Boy George. Many of the members had and were curious about his sound. So I played some of his music, and it turned out to be a hit with them. Similarly, the group became breakdance music and "rappin'" fans when breakdancers put on a show in their cafeteria.

In short, the use of music can enhance the geriatric fitness student's experience as long as it doesn't become the central focus of meetings. Nursing homes usually have music and sing-along classes for that. So pay attention to how music affects your group's participation levels, and adjust its use accordingly. In other words, keeping in mind the ultimate goals of your program, play it by ear!

A Bulletin Board for Motivation

If a real cork bulletin board is not available, a large piece of poster paper works fine as a focal point on which to tape photographs and other materials related to fitness class.

The board should be labelled with large, clear letters. For this, you can use a wide felt-tipped marker or pre-cut press-on letters, which are sold by the package in office supply stores.

You may want to hold a group discussion to decide on the wording of your bulletin board's title. Does the group already have an official name? If not, the members can agree on one which can then be used on the board. Be prepared to make name suggestions yourself, but use members' ideas when possible in order to promote a feeling of involvement among your students. People tend to care most about programs that they have had a part in shaping.

Make a special event out of starting a bulletin board by displaying it to your class and by explaining what it is for. Let them watch or help as you mount it in its permanent location on the wall. On an ongoing basis, new items to be featured on the board can be passed around, discussed, and then posted during meetings.

The bulletin board should be located within view of the group circle and in a well-travelled part of the nursing home. This way, members frequently get to see pictures of themselves which were taken during class. Non-members see, too, and may become interested enough to try the class. A good bulletin board can help to keep fitness class on the residents' minds and in their conversations.

Most nursing homes keep a camera, and the activities coordinator can arrange for occasional photographs to be taken during your meetings.

Turn Your Students into Celebrities

Newspaper clippings make even better bulletin board material. I'm not talking about health articles cut out of the newspaper, although some of

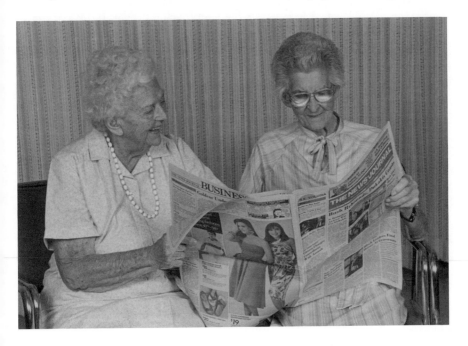

those may be appropriate, too. I mean news stories about your particular fitness group!

So give your students a claim to fame. Notify local news publications when you are planning a special event (such as the multi-sport wheelchair competition that is described in Chapter Four). Often the editor will dispatch a photographer to capture the story on film.

Your activities coordinator has probably invited members of the local media to the home before. If so, the coordinator may already know editors and reporters well enough to make the contact for you. Do make a point not to call on the local press too frequently and not to ask them for coverage of trivial, unnewsworthy events. They will remain receptive to your news items if you invite them to special occasions that are likely to be of interest to the general community.

Your Monthly Newsletter: Another Motivator

Many nursing homes distribute a monthly newsletter to residents and staff. In many cases, this is a shoestring operation with news being gathered by activities personnel and typed onto standard white 8½ x 11 paper, then printed by a copier machine in the business office. The pages may then be stapled together at the top left corner, or they may be folded and stapled in the center to form a booklet. Personnel in charge of a nursing home newsletter are almost always eager for contributions, even tidbits of news, to include.

As group fitness leader, you can utilize such a publication to generate support for your work among the nursing home's staff and administration. When they have some understanding of exactly what it is you do, aids may be more willing to help certain residents get up and ready in time for morning fitness meetings. Administrators may be more willing to authorize expenditures for balls, chalk, records, or tape cassettes.

Relatives of the residents often receive newsletters, and this presents you with an opportunity to promote your fitness program to people who can be instrumental in encouraging residents to attend class. For example, a visiting daughter may barely be aware that a fitness program exists until she picks up a copy of the newsletter. But when she reads about the fun and progress that other residents are enjoying in the class, she may want the same benefits for her mother. Then she will begin actively urging her mother to participate.

For your students, the newsletter represents positive fitness reinforcement. Seeing their names in print alongside a recap of their accomplishments affords a reward for their efforts. They can be proud to enclose copies of the news in with letters they write to distant loved ones. They will be able to tell of interesting and current achievements to their visitors. As each month's issue is published, they will enjoy having their new fitness report read aloud during class. By doing this, you can also make sure that students mentioned by name know they are featured in the newsletter and that everyone has received a copy of his own.

Special activities in which the group takes part can be written up in paragraph form. Below are some representative examples of fitness news items that can be written up in list form:

MARY JONES deserves special recognition for fitness class attendance. She didn't miss a meeting during the whole month of January!

ALBERT BISHOP made ten perfect kicks in a row during our ball game last Monday.

MARGARET ADAMS shared a funny yarn about the time her dog stole a pie from the windowsill during one of our group discussions.

FRANCES SMITH and ANNA BAKER both became members of our fitness group in January. Welcome!

More examples of typical fitness group news items are included at the end of this chapter.

As you can see, it only takes ten or fifteen minutes per month to jot down a few interesting notes about recent fitness gatherings. Remember to ask your students, too, for ideas about news they'd like to see included.

Printing a student's name in bold face or capital letters makes it easy for him to spot it and, at the same time, lends additional importance to his news.

In fact, try to make your whole report easy to read. Most folks of any age are more likely to read a short write-up than a lengthy one. Double-spacing the lines will be a help to weak eyes. If you write in a simple style using short, clear sentences, you will attract more readers — not only from among the residents, but from the staff as well.

If your nursing home's newsletter is a low-budget operation, you can type the report yourself and turn it in ready to print. If you are turning in a handwritten report or if all contributions are routinely retyped before layout, just attach a note requesting a double-spaced, easy-to-read format.

One way to draw attention to your fitness news is to supply an illustration to go with it. At the end of this chapter, you will find twelve pictures, one for each monthly report during the year.

Using a black felt-tipped pen, trace the picture onto plain white typewriter paper. If the report you turn in is to be run as is, leave space to trace the picture where you want it to appear on the same sheet that you type on. If your report is to be retyped before publication, trace it onto a separate sheet of clean white paper and turn it in with your text sheet.

The illustrations included at the end of this chapter are very simple line drawings so that they can be quickly and easily traced and so that any kind of copier machine should be able to reproduce them clearly. If your nursing home's newsletter is a technically advanced production, you may be able to use more elaborate artwork with your reports. Discuss this with the staff member in charge of putting the publication together.

If your nursing home does not sponsor a monthly newsletter, consider using the ideas and diagrams in this chapter to produce a one-page fitness letter of your own each month. It wouldn't take much effort or time to type a few double-spaced lines of news and to trace on a picture at the bottom of the page. The nursing home can probably provide for the copying.

In brief, as a geriatric fitness leader, you'll want to use every tool available to you that might help to inspire fitness class attendance and participation.

Encouragement: The Ultimate Key to Success

In writing this chapter, I have tried to include considerations that are important in the management of fitness groups composed of elderly students. But none of the factors discussed before is as essential as the one I have saved for last: encouragement. Praise is required to elicit prolonged effort from the elderly — not frivolous, meaningless flattery (they will see through that in a minute), but deserved recognition for real effort made.

Many students may be frustrated by their disabilities or sadly aware of physical capacities that have diminished dramatically since youth. Sometimes they may feel depressed or even bitter because they cannot run, leap, kick, and brawl like they could in times long past. You have an opportunity to help these persons to feel vital, competent, and successful once more. And sure enough, as they begin to enjoy these feelings again, they *will* be more vital, competent, and successful.

With that in mind, use encouragement even when students fail. For example, if someone misses a catch, be sure to say, "Good try!"

A few more exclamations that a leader should keep ready on the tongue are: *good job, good going, perfect, super, terrific, excellent, all right, that's the way,* and *now you're doing it!* Pepper your class with these encouragements, and watch each student to make sure he earns at least one during every meeting. You will soon be well on the way to developing a willing, responsive group. Try combining encouragement with other motivators, such as calling your students by name. "Real good, Sarah" accompanied by a pat on the back can work wonders on a student's energy level.

Always remember that in order to achieve an optimistic, can-do atmosphere, you've got to let your students know that you believe in them and their abilities.

In Summary

Dealing successfully with a group of elderly students boils down to supporting them, treating them with dignity, and respecting them as the adult human beings that they are.

If you expect elderly people to work for you, and a fitness leader *must* expect this, you have to give them a reason to work. From the start, you must get along with them well. And ultimately, you must gain their trust by demonstrating that you truly care.

If you feel that these abilities are not part of your nature, perhaps you should leave geriatric fitness instruction to others. But please don't sell yourself short. If you possess that basic quality — caring — you can work at practicing the do's and don't's we have discussed in this chapter. Before long, you will grow comfortable with these principles, and you will be ready to meet the challenge.

SUPPLEMENT A

Typical examples of fitness-related news appropriate for contribution to nursing home newsletter:

CAROLYN BOLT's daughter Amy attended fitness class as her mother's guest.

JOHN ADAMS and BETH WILLIAMS are both able to touch their toes now!

ANDREW HUNT won the wheelchair race on Thursday. ALMA ANDERSON came in second place, and LAURA MASON came in third.

BECKY SHARP told the best riddle during group discussion. Ask her about it!

JIM PAGE asked us to cut short our discussion of the recent Bethune Beach picnic. He said we were making him hungry!

BILL BRADFORD and his family agree that he is walking better since he began attending fitness class.

HELEN CALDWELL kicked the beach ball all the way out of the cafeteria.

BEA ROGERS says she especially enjoyed our outdoor fitness meeting last month.

MILDRED BARNES correctly showed our group where the biceps muscle is located.

BOB MILLER's folks have given him a foam ball to squeeze in his room on days when fitness group doesn't meet.

ALL OF US thoroughly enjoyed playing dodge ball with BRYAN and CINDY MARTIN, preteen children of staff member, WILMA MARTIN, R.N.

CHUCK BEATTY told some hilarious tales about all the monkey-business he got into as a youngster and had us all in stitches during group discussion.

JEAN LANDERS correctly demonstrated how to do the "row boat" exercise.

MARY JONES and MARGARET ADAMS are improving their kickball skills at every meeting.

ANNA BAKER appeared in class wearing a lovely new pink bathrobe which was a gift from her son and which was admired by all present.

SUPPLEMENT B

One-year supply of simple diagrams suitable for tracing onto monthly fitness reports:

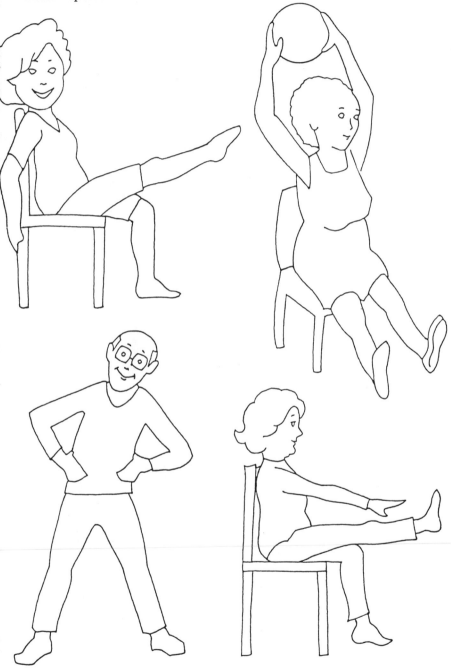

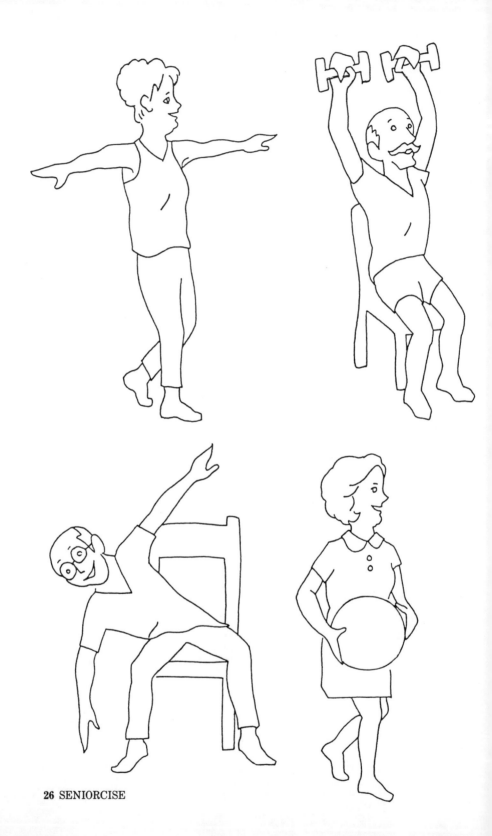

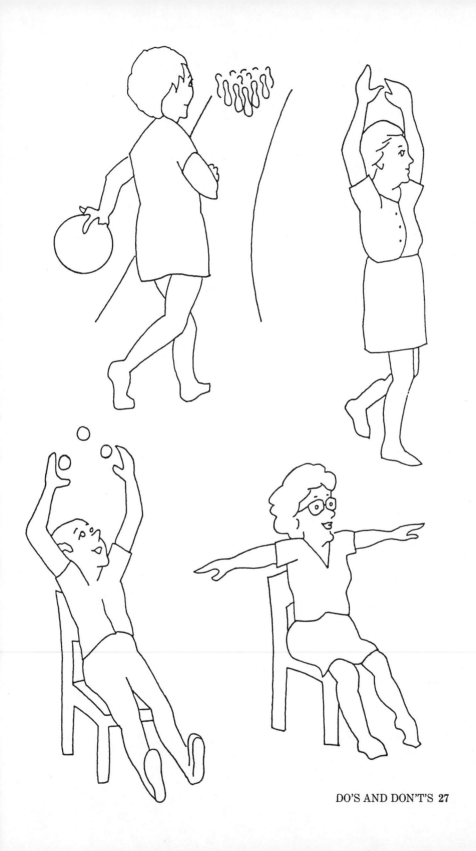

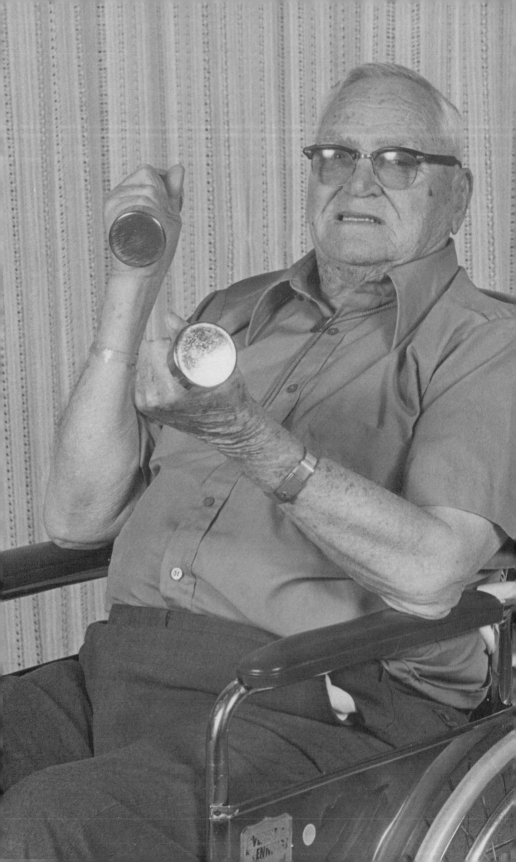

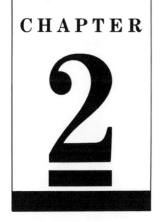

CHAPTER 2

Sit-Down Workouts from Head to Toe

Goals: Mobility, Grip, Strength and Flexibility

The specific objectives of Seniorcise are quite different from those of a health club aerobics program, in which members seek better figures and cardiovascular training. The retiree resident is well served by exercises aimed at maintaining joint mobility, which is important when it comes to steering one's wheelchair or continuing to get about on foot. He benefits from gripping exercises which foster the ability to hang onto coffee mugs, eating utensils, hair brushes, and pencils. Flexibility and strength are also worthwhile goals. In fact, one of my students came to class glowing with pride when she regained the capability to maneuver herself without aid from her bed to her wheelchair and back.

Typically, a nursing home resident who joins the Seniorcise program will soon report that he is beginning to feel more energetic. His muscle tone and coordination skills stand to improve as well. All of these factors can play a big role in making his everyday life more manageable and enjoyable.

Concerning Aerobics

In the simplest terms, aerobic exercise contributes toward physical fitness by placing a demand upon the heart muscle. In order to be effective, the aerobic effort must meet specific requisites with regard to intensity, duration, and frequency. It is a relatively strenuous type of exercise.

Although it is possible to achieve aerobic conditioning when exercising in a wheelchair, this book will not give instructions for aerobic workouts. Remember that we are dealing with the very elderly, some of whom have seen an entire century! The brisk, continuous arm motions that are required to elevate the heart rate (when a person is seated in a chair) call for strength and endurance that most nursing home residents do not possess. Although greater strength and endurance can be developed gradually, there are other problems to consider.

During aerobics, some students will not be able to pace themselves properly by counting their pulse rates or by following Borg's Relative Perceived Exertion Scale, a subjective method of pacing.

Furthermore, it is important that all nursing home residents be stress tested before engaging in aerobic exercise. This testing will have to be modified to accommodate students who cannot use their legs and for students with high blood pressure, diabetes, arthritis, and other special conditions. Most nursing homes do not have sufficient resources to engage the professional supervision and equipment necessary for these essential testing procedures.

No one should supervise aerobic exercise for students of *any* age without training in CPR (cardiopulmonary resuscitation) in addition to certification in aerobic exercise instruction by a reputable agency such as The Aerobics and Fitness Association of America. Due to the medical histories of the students involved, an instructor of group aerobics in a nursing home environment should acquire further in-depth and specialized training. If members of your group do progress to the level of sustaining continuous energetic arm movements for twenty to thirty consecutive minutes — *and* if your nursing home supports the idea of having an aerobics program *and* if it has the wherewithal to secure suitable stress testing for your students — consider obtaining appropriate certification. For more information, you can contact The Aerobics and Fitness Association of America, 15250 Ventura Boulevard, Suite 310, Sherman Oaks, California 91403.

Because aerobic work produces desirable training effects (such as conditioning the cardiovascular system, enhancing the body's fat-to-lean-mass ratio, and improving serum cholesterol levels), it is widely accepted as the most beneficial form of physical exercise. In fact, some nursing home students do reap the profits of performing aerobic activity. In responsible programs of this nature, trained personnel carefully and continuously monitor the participants, and the rewards are very, very great. But I would strongly caution you against launching an aerobic exercise program for nursing home residents without the total commitment and permanent involvement of a qualified medical team.

Getting Started

Without extensive testing, nursing home staff physicians can provide written clearance for residents to enroll in light, general exercise courses such as the one described in this book. After your membership is established, you can apply the following principles to help each individual gain his most from the group workout.

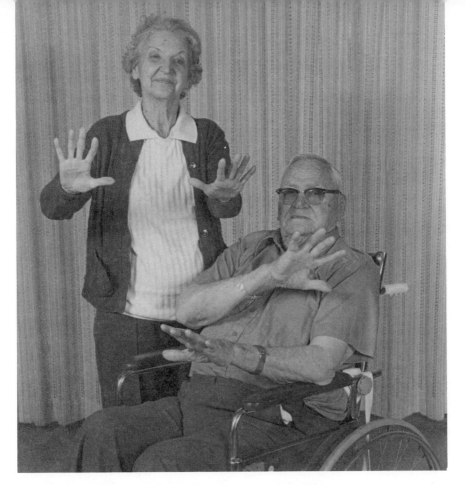

Exercising While Standing, Sitting, or Lying Down

Since many of your members will be confined to wheelchairs and even ambulatory members may tire easily, all exercises should be achievable from the seated position. Never remove seat belts or other forms of restraint, even when a student argues eloquently for release. You can, however, ask an aid or nurse to check a restraint if it appears uncomfortably tight. Make certain that wheelchair brakes are set so that chairs do not roll during the exercise session. And, allow plenty of space between chairs in your group circle so that students will have enough room to perform their arm work.

Stronger members may enjoy standing through some of the exercises, for example during arm scissors and biceps curls. While performing these arm motions they can stand still, or shift their hips from side to side, or walk in place in rhythm with the primary motions (or with musical accompaniment, if used). To protect the spine when standing, knees should be slightly bent, never locked. The back should be straight, not swayed. To improve balance when legs are stationary, the feet should be placed apart at a distance equal to shoulder width, and the body's weight should be evenly distributed over both legs. If a standing student shows signs of fatigue, have him retire to his seat where he can continue to exercise.

These standing modifications are particularly appropriate for members who are considerably younger than most of the other nursing home residents. One of my students, only in her mid-sixties, lives in the nursing home because she has Alzheimer's disease. On most days she has no problem following the workout and, in fact, likes the added challenge of performing some of the exercises while standing.

On the other side of the coin, many of the exercises included in this chapter can be performed while lying or sitting up in bed. All of the facial, hand, and wrist exercises can be done lying down. Almost all of the arm movements can be done lying or sitting. Most of the head, neck, and shoulder movements can be done while propped up on a pillow. And the toe point/flex and ankle rotation exercises can be done from any position.

Breathing Easy

Members should receive frequent reminders to breathe steadily and regularly during exercise. Sometimes an exerciser will concentrate so hard on the specific move he is trying to execute that he may hold his breath without even realizing he's doing it. By the same token, don't be offended if a member begins to yawn during your workout. His body is simply responding to exertion by asking for extra oxygen.

And-a-One-and-a-Two

Counting exercise repetitions aloud helps students to pace themselves, and some will enjoy counting along with you. "Count-downs" (counting the repetitions backwards to zero) add fun and variety to the workout and, at the same time, make pacing even easier. Be sure to state in advance of each exercise exactly how many repetitions are to be performed. But do not confuse your nursing home students by counting in sets. Sets are good in classes for the general public. An instructor may say, "We're going to do four sets of eight," and then count like this: *1*2345678, *2*2345678, *3*2345678, and so on. In nursing home group class it is better to say, "We're going to do twenty of these," and then to count out twenty repetitions, either forwards or backwards.

Pumping Iron

Some members will be able to utilize handweights during class, and this is one effective way to strengthen muscles. Canned goods straight from the kitchen cabinet make fine equipment. The exact weight of every can is stated on its label. Members can begin with single-serving sizes, which are extremely light, and work their way up to heavier weights. For the member

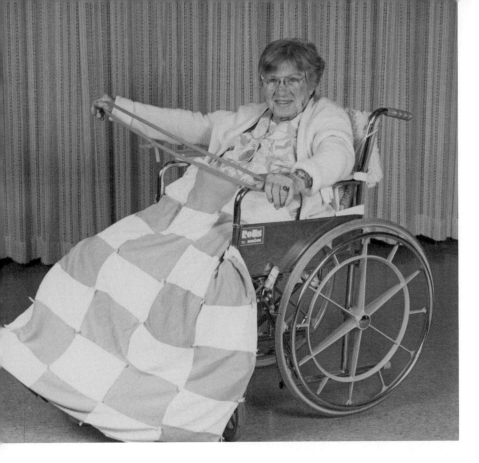

who needs help with gripping, the can may be slipped inside an ordinary sock, which is then knotted at the open end. This provides an easy-to-grip texture. As you study the exercise workouts provided later in this chapter, note that many of the arm movements can be performed while holding handweights. You can utilize your nursing home newsletter (or a bulletin board in the employee break room) to ask staff members to donate canned goods for the "gym."

Accessories

Of course, you can also purchase more sophisticated means of resistance. It is not imperative that you do so, and, in fact, the cost may be prohibitive. You should, however, be aware that additional options are available.

Medical supply catalogs feature exercise aids that are often ordered by physical therapy departments. Thera-Plast, for example, is a putty-like substance useful for grip-type exercise. And Thera-Band, a strip of material with texture similar to that of a balloon, can be tied to wheelchair arms or bed rails for push and pull exercise.

For details on these products you can contact Fred Sammons, Inc.,

A Bissell Healthcare Co., Box 32, Brookfield, IL. 60513-0032 (1-800-323-5547). The physical therapy department and medical supply office of your nursing home will probably be able to recommend additional products and distributors.

Your medical supply office can also order soft surgical tubing, which can be cut into three-foot lengths and tied at the ends to form bungie cords. At approximately twenty dollars per fifty feet, this makes an economical material for push-pull exercise.

Keep It Cool
Exercise should never be executed with fast or jerky motions or with joints locked rigidly. Instead, demonstrate the moves using a slow to moderate speed. Keep movements gentle, deliberate, and smooth.

Stress Signals
A student should stop exercising and rest if he experiences any of the following symptoms:

- lightheadedness,
- shortness of breath,
- over-fatigue.

The student should stop exercising and you should alert medical staff immediately if he experiences any of the following symptoms:

- dizziness,
- severe shortness of breath,
- chest pain,
- sharp pain anywhere,
- shakiness or trembling,
- queasiness or nausea,
- throbbing head,
- any sensation of an unusual or questionable character.

Do not rely solely on the student to keep you posted on how he is feeling. Do observe the members of your group closely at all times. Be on the lookout for signs of stress. If a situation ever occurs in which you are not sure whether or not you should call a nurse, do it.

What's the Point?
Nursing home students exercise more willingly when the activities make sense to them. For that reason, remember to explain the purpose of the

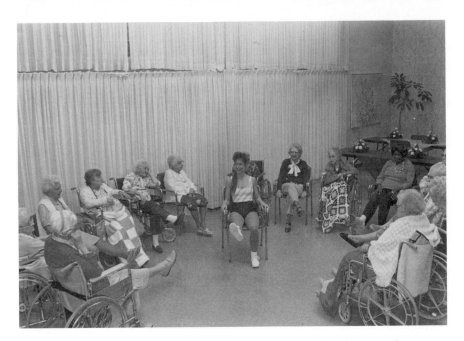

movement you are proposing. Examples: "This exercise helps to keep your shoulder joints mobile. I like to think of it as oiling my joints so that they won't get rusty." "Being flexible is handy when it comes to putting on your sweater." "Stretching helps to prevent stiffness in your joints and cramps in your muscles." "Moving your trunk is especially beneficial if you do a lot of sitting, since shifting your weight relieves pressure." "Exercising your arms gives them extra strength for powering that wheelchair."

From Top to Bottom

Along those same lines, my nursing home students appreciate the logic and flow of workouts that follow an orderly progression. Jumping around from shoulder work to leg work, back up to neck work, and then down to foot work will make it more difficult for them to pace themselves, because they won't have a good feel for how far along they are in the whole workout. Physically, it is beneficial to exercise muscles or groups of muscles long enough for them to feel tired. The workouts described in this chapter, then, will exercise the body starting at the top and working downward. Be careful, however, not to exhaust students, causing them to drop out of the workout before completion. If your students look fatigued or complain of feeling tired before you have finished with one particular area, you may move on to the next area, then come back and finish the first after the tired muscles have had a chance to rest.

As a matter of fact, when you are working with new students, you need not have them try to perform every exercise listed here for a given area. Try a progressive approach instead. For example, the upper body section of each workout includes many exercises. You can teach new students a few of the exercises at your first meeting, then add one or two additional exercises at each subsequent meeting. This gives students time to build up strength and to become familiar with the exercises gradually.

Coping with Disease

A wide range of restrictive diseases can exist among the members of one nursing home fitness group. Students should be encouraged to do as much of the exercise as they can, but to stop and to tell you if they experience pain. If this occurs, you should notify nursing home medical staff.

Most diseases are self-restrictive. For example, you need only to reassure the student with a leg amputation that he can still excel at exercises using his other leg and his arms. In order to avoid unnecessary irritation, do check the stump now and then to make sure that there is no excess rubbing of the skin against wheelchair or prosthesis.

Students with certain conditions such as multiple sclerosis, stroke, or cerebral palsy may experience coordination problems. Changing quickly from one exercise movement to another will be extremely difficult for them. So, do allow ample transition time between changes, and then do allow them plenty of time with each motion once they've mastered it, before they have to move on to another.

Additional considerations are in order for the stroke victim. If exercise is too vigorous, his joints may be strained and he will experience pain. So, again, let me stress the importance of exercising with smooth, gentle motions. If he already suffers from pain, it will prevail as a self-limiting element during exercise. So, don't be demanding — be encouraging.

When a stroke patient is paralyzed on one side of his body he will be able to perform better in fitness class if his unimpaired side is nearer the action. Although one stroke patient may tend to neglect his impaired side altogether, another may learn to use his strong limb to help the weaker one complete some of the exercise movements.

If a stroke patient is paralyzed on his right side he may have special problems related to communication. If so, he will probably be more successful in fitness class if you demonstrate exercises for him instead of giving verbal instructions. In conversation, you can help him by keeping your speech patterns short, simple, and to the point.

If paralyzed on the left side, a stroke patient may have trouble with *spatial-perceptual* values such as size, position, and rate of speed. For example, it may be hard for him to distinguish right from left or to judge the distance between himself and another person or object. Try not to overwhelm him with quick movements and gestures. Although he might not be able to duplicate an exercise that you demonstrate, he may be able to do it if you give him verbal instructions.

The polio victim is likely to encounter self-restricting muscle atrophy along with a considerable reduction in the range of motion of his joints. Remember that his best version of the specific exercise you are leading is always acceptable and praiseworthy.

The same rule applies to students with emphysema, cardiovascular disease, and inoperable malignant tumors. Even though all of your students have been given medical permission to exercise, those with certain chronic conditions may become tired and winded easily. Let them do as much light exercise as they feel capable of. Reward their efforts with appropriate recognition. Do not push or prod them into over-exertion.

The diabetic is a very special exerciser indeed and may require extra medical attention in connection with his workout. If he receives an insulin shot immediately before exercise, the injection site should be an area of the body that will not be worked. If his speech becomes slurred or if he appears confused or bewildered during exercise, stop the exercise and call for medical aid at once. He may be experiencing exercise-engendered hypoglycemia. Other signals to watch out for are hunger and profuse perspiration. If hypoglycemia is induced, medical staff will probably administer sugar. In fact, modifications in insulin dosage and/or diet can prevent it from occurring. These, however, are medical decisions, not fitness decisions. I have never had any diabetic student to encounter a complication during Seniorcise, and you should not expect problems. However, should one arise, you should be aware of the information above in order to be able to work cooperatively with medical staff.

The student with rheumatoid arthritis may suffer from joint damage. Avoid sustaining any single, fixed exercise position for very long at a time. Advocate good posture. Respect the fact that disease-induced deformities (especially in hands and feet) will be self-limiting elements during exercise. In other words, don't ever force the issue with a body by asking it to do something it *will not*. This student may, by the way, perform better during afternoon classes since stiffness is usually more pronounced in the morning.

The student with a permanent injury to his spine may have no movement or function in either leg. He may exhibit muscle atrophy and range of motion limitation as well as the tendency to fatigue easily. He may have trouble maintaining an upright seated position. He should be encouraged to execute the exercises from which he is not self-limited. However, his lower back should not be stretched, and he should not sit in exactly the same position for more than approximately fifteen minutes at a time with no shift in weight and pressure. There are many different types of spinal column injuries. If you have a student with spinal injury, you should ask his physician for a list of exercise do's and don't's specific to his particular condition.

Blindness may result from various disorders, including diabetes. The student with an eye-related disability should not be asked to nod low at the front or to lean forward so far that his head falls below chest level. The purpose behind these exceptions is to prevent unnecessary blood flow or pressure to the eyes. He can perform a shallow version of these movements or simply enjoy a "rest set" during their execution. In the beginning of a fitness program, it may be helpful to the blind student to manually guide him through the exercises. Use a light, gentle touch while respecting his self-limitations and natural range of motion. Later on, he will be able to recognize the exercises from your descriptions and will require little or no hands-on assistance.

We have discussed some of the physical disorders most commonly found among nursing home fitness class students. Remember that some students will have tender spots on problem feet or fingers, and some may be sore from recent surgical procedures. Some will wear catheters or nasal prongs. So be careful never to bump or jar these delicate areas.

Caution with Necks

Exercises that mildly stretch the neck bring pleasure to many nursing home students and help them to feel limber. However, extra caution should be taken when performing any movement that affects the neck. Neck exercises must be executed with gentleness and moderation. The circling motions described in the neck section of Seniorcise Workout 1 should be carried out slowly and should involve small circles, not head rolls. Some students will be able to achieve greater stability and control by keeping their shoulders slightly elevated when they move their heads.

Students with inner ear disorders should forego the neck exercises. As I mentioned earlier, sight-disabled students should not nod too low at the front. Certain other students, such as stroke patients, could run into trouble controlling their movements during the exercises, which would make them injury prone. So if a student's head tends to roll or if his motions appear "floppy," then excuse him from participating in the neck exercises. If several members of the group have trouble controlling these exercises, then omit the neck section from the workout entirely. Compensate by doing more of the other stretches your students find pleasant and refreshing.

When in Doubt

Most importantly, remember that the nursing home's medical team is a fitness instructor's invaluable ally. Show consideration for their time by approaching them in a professional manner with succinct, well-thought-out inquiries. If you have questions regarding a particular exercise, call on the physical therapist. If you have questions regarding a particular student,

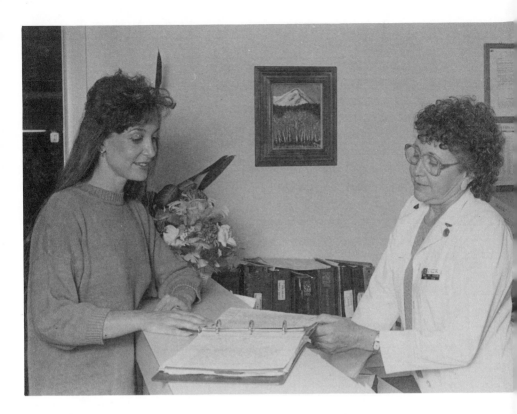

consult his nurse or physician.

OK, now that we've addressed the theory associated with nursing home exercise, let's move on to the workouts!

The Workouts

When you begin working with a new nursing home fitness class, use the lowest number of repetitions listed. As your members become stronger and more accustomed to the exercises, add more repetitions. When possible, increase the number by increments of five, so that the number of repetitions will be easy for students to remember (for instance: five, ten, or fifteen). On certain exercises, you may eventually want to exceed the maximum number of repetitions I have listed. However, it will take months of working with the same students to reach that point. By that time, you will know your group's abilities and limitations very well and should be able to judge how many repetitions the members can handle. Where exercise performance is timed by the passage of seconds, the numbers are intended as general guides to you as the leader. With a little practice, you will be able to approximate these times mentally and, therefore, should never have to invest in a stopwatch.

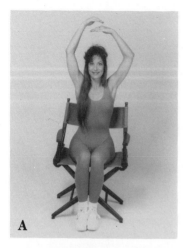

A

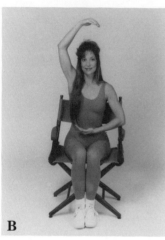

B

Posture/Breathing:

1) Sit up straight. Encourage students to use the best seated posture possible.

2) Breathe in and out slowly and deeply. Three times.

3) Breathe in and out slowly and deeply along with "ballet" arm motions. As you inhale, raise both arms up in a high arc. As you exhale, lower arms in an arc to chest level. Encourage students to be very graceful, like a ballerina. Three times. **A**

4) Breathe in and out slowly and deeply along with alternate "ballet" arm motions. As you inhale, raise one arm up in an arc. As you exhale, lower it in an arc. Repeat using other arm and continue alternating. Four times (two per arm); work up to six times (three per arm). **B**

Face:

1) Open and close your eyes. Five times; work up to ten.

2) Open and close your mouth. Five times; work up to ten.

Neck:

1) Slowly lean one ear downward toward shoulder and relax there for three seconds. Raise head to the center, then lean other ear downward toward opposite shoulder and relax there for three seconds. Alternate. Six times (three per side).

2) Slowly lower chin toward chest and relax there for three seconds, then raise head high enough to look straight ahead and hold for three seconds. Do not exaggerate this motion by looking straight up and leaning the head back, as that may compress vertebrae in the upper spine. Alternate. Six times (three each way).

3) Circle head in small, slow circles. This motion should be executed gently and conservatively. Five times in one direction, then five in the opposite direction.

Upper Body (Shoulder Girdle/Upper Arms):

1) Shrug both shoulders up and down at a moderate speed. Ten times; work up to fifteen.

2) Alternate shoulder shrugs. Ten times (five per side); work up to twenty.

3) Interlock fingers in front of chest. Raise hands as high as possible and then lower them behind the head. Three times; work up to five. **A,B,C**

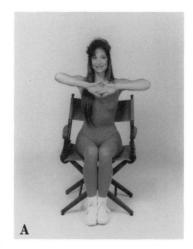

A

4) Start with arms bent at sides, elbows at shoulder level, and hands in front of chest. At a moderate speed, press elbows backwards. Return to starting position. Ten times; work up to twenty. **D**

5) Clap hands together in front of chest. Twenty times.

6) Clap hands together high over head. Twenty times.

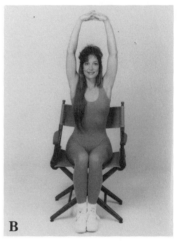

B

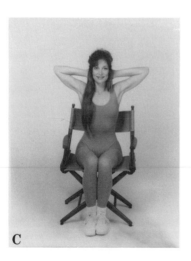

C

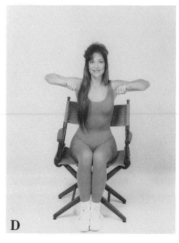

D

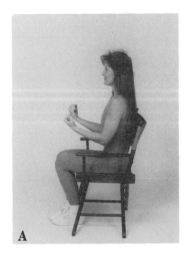

A

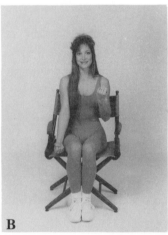

B

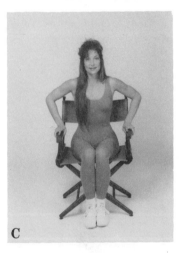

C

7) Biceps curls: With elbows fixed low at sides, curl your forearms at a moderate speed upward to the front while flexing the biceps muscle. Then lower the forearms. Encourage students to "squeeze up," to "flex," to "contract," to "use the muscleman muscle" (point to it). Ten times; work up to fifteen. **A**

8) Alternate biceps curls: Same as above, except that as one forearm is lowered the other is raised. Ten times (five curls per arm); work up to twenty. **B**

9) Pushups: With elbows bent, grasp the arms of the chair with your hands. Using the muscles in your arms, push down in order to raise the body upward at a moderate speed. As your body rises, both arms should become straighter (but not straight enough to lock the elbow joints). Ease back into starting position. The stronger student will be able to lift his buttocks clear of the chair's seat. Check the ambulatory student to make sure he is not using legs and feet to elevate his body. If he is, have him cross his ankles, lift feet off the floor, and hold. Have him perform the pushups while holding feet up in order to ensure that he uses his arms to execute the lifts. Three times; work up to ten. **C,D**

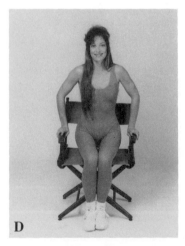

D

10) Extend arms at sides. At a moderate speed, make small circles forward using the entire arm. Five times; work up to fifteen.

11) Same as above, except circle backwards. Five times; work up to fifteen.

12) Extend arms to the front at shoulder level. At a moderate speed, make small circles in one direction using the entire arm. Five times; work up to fifteen.

13) Same as above, except circle in the opposite direction. Five times; work up to fifteen.

14) With hands flexed, push both arms up high over head at a moderately slow speed. Lower both to lap. Five times; work up to fifteen. **A,B**

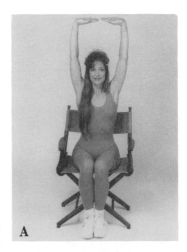

A

15) Same as above, except push out to the front at chest level. Five times; work up to fifteen.

16) Military press: Start with arms bent at sides, elbows at shoulder level, palms facing the front. Extend both arms upward. Return to starting position. Five times; work up to fifteen. **C,D**

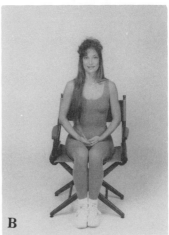

B

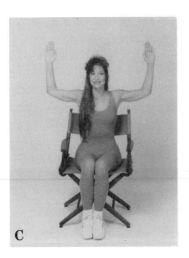

C

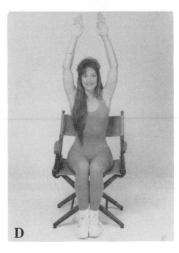

D

Wrists:

1) With fingers straight, move hands at a moderate speed in a circular pattern at the wrists. Make certain that students move hands only, not arms. Ten revolutions.

2) Same as above, except circle in the opposite direction. Ten revolutions.

Forearms/Hands/Fingers:

1) Make a tight fist, then spread fingers wide. Alternate. Ten times (ten fisted, ten spread); work up to twenty.

2) Wriggle fingers vigorously (fingers only, not hands or arms). Continue for thirty seconds to one minute.

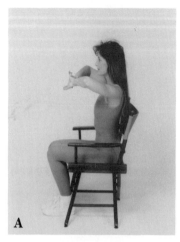

A

3) Interlock fingers in front of chest. Turn palms outward towards the front. At a moderately slow speed, extend arms forward until fingers feel stretched. Five times; work up to ten. **A,B**

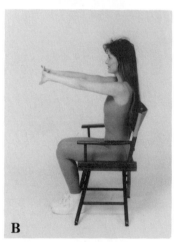

B

Abdomen:

1) When one is contraindicated from performing situps and crunches, it is difficult to exercise the abdomen adequately. The following exercise will put abdominal muscle to work for the person in a seated or lying position. It does, however, require concentration on the part of the exerciser. So a scenario was devised to help the student focus on the area to be exercised:

"Envision yourself in a swimsuit on the beach. To your surprise, along comes Marilyn Monroe or Cary Grant. What will you tend to do while your idol has you in view? Suck in that tummy and hold it as flat as possible, that's what! Hold it in — he's still looking — keep it flat (two to three seconds). OK, he has passed. You can relax now (five to ten seconds). But look! Here comes Sophia Loren or Clark Gable. We'd better pull those stomachs in flat again. Hold it in . . ." And so on. Two times; work up to five.

Caution the students that just because they are holding in their stomachs this does not mean that they should hold in their breath, too. Remind them during each hold to breathe naturally.

Waist:

1) With your arms resting lightly on the arms of the chair, gently turn your torso towards one side and then the other. Six times (three each way); work up to ten.

2) Start from the same position as above. Circle your torso in gentle revolutions. Five times in one direction; five times in the opposite direction; work up to ten.

Buttocks:

1) The same principle as that used for the abdomen applies to the buttocks. Have the student shift his focus to his buttocks. Concentrate, squeeze (two to three seconds), then release. Rest for a few seconds before repeating. If a scenario is needed to help the student isolate the correct muscles, you can continue the story from above: "Now Robert Mitchum is standing behind you, and you know he's looking. Tighten up that bottom!" Two times; work up to five.

Lower Back:

1) Sit with feet flat on floor or wheel-chair footrests. Slowly allow the upper body to fall forward from the hips as far as feels natural and comfortable. Consciously relax in that position with arms hanging loose at the sides. Head, neck, and shoulders should be free of any tension or rigidity. Remain in this position for a few seconds (if comfortable). Then slowly raise back up to an upright position. As you rise, try to keep arms, head, neck, and shoulders as relaxed as possible. Remain upright for five to ten seconds before repeating. Three times; work up to five.

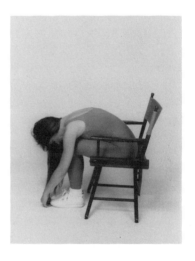

Many nursing home students will not be able to stretch downward very far. They should be encouraged to lean forward just far enough to feel a pleasant stretch. Those who are restrained by ties or seatbelts will be in no danger of falling too far. Those without restraints should be instructed to watch their balance, leaning forward and downward only as far as they feel secure.

Upper Legs:

1) Use your hands to rub and massage the front of your legs at and above

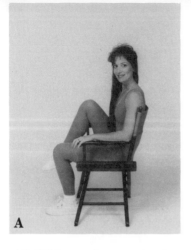

A

the knees. Thirty seconds to one minute.

2) "Walk" in place while seated. Thirty seconds to one minute.

3) "March" in place while seated. Thirty seconds to one minute.

4) Alternate bent knee lifts. Ten times (five per leg); work up to twenty. **A**

5) Lift one leg, which has been straightened just short of locking the knee. Ten times; then lift the other leg ten times; work up to fifteen.

6) With one foot on the floor, extend the other leg and straighten it just short of locking the knee. At a moderately slow speed, complete five large circles in one direction using the entire leg. Then complete five circles in the opposite direction. Repeat using the other leg. Work up from five to ten circles each way.

Nursing home students follow this exercise particularly well when you count forward during the first five circles and backwards during the next five, which are towards the opposite direction.

Ankles:

1) Extend both legs and rotate your feet in circles at the ankle. Do not rotate or swing your legs. Ten rotations in one direction; ten in the opposite direction.

Lower Legs/Feet/Toes:

1) Alternate pointing your toes and flexing your feet. Twenty times (ten points, ten flexes); work up to forty. **B,C**

My nursing home students enjoy referring to this activity as more of their "ballet" exercise. A good variation of this exercise is to alternate pointing one side while flexing the other.

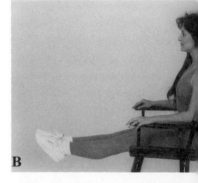

B

Relaxation:

1) Close your eyes and repeat "ballet-style" deep breathing exercises from the Posture/Breathing section, except perform all more slowly and very luxuriously.

2) With eyes still closed, give yourself a gentle hug, then relax. Three times.

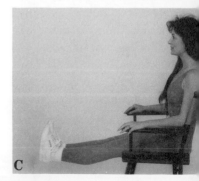

C

Seniorcise Workout 2

Begin your routine with the same Posture/Breathing exercises outlined in Seniorcise Workout 1. These basic exercises are the starters for all Seniorcise workouts, and your students will respond well to beginning each workout on a familiar note.

Face:

1) Assume facial expressions which reflect the following moods: happy, sad, amused, surprised, and angry.

This is an exercise that you and your students can have a lot of fun with. Think of other feelings that can be depicted with facial expressions, and ask your students to suggest new feelings to be expressed.

Neck:

1) Say "Yes." Gently nod at a moderate speed for thirty seconds.

2) Say "No." Gently turn your head at a moderate speed for thirty seconds.

3) Say "Maybe." Gently alternate tilting your head from side to side for thirty seconds.

Upper Body (Shoulder Girdle/Upper Arms):

1) Circle both shoulders forward. Five times; work up to ten.

2) Alternate circling one shoulder forward and then the other. Ten times (five per shoulder); work up to twenty.

3) Same as Exercise #1 above, except circle backwards. Five times; work up to ten.

4) Same as Exercise #2 above, except circle backwards. Ten times (five per shoulder); work up to twenty.

5) Arm scissors: With palms facing down and hands and fingers straight, criss-cross the arms back and forth at chest level. Thirty seconds; work up to one minute.

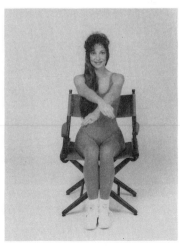

6) Still scissoring as above, raise and lower arms as high and as low as possible at the front. Thirty seconds; work up to one minute.

7) Same as Exercise #5 above, except with palms facing up. Thirty seconds; work up to one minute.

8) Same as Exercise #6 above, except with palms facing up. Thirty seconds; work up to one minute.

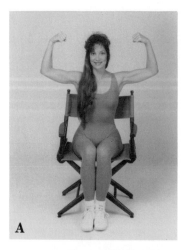

A

9) Slow biceps curls: With arms extended to the sides at shoulder level, slowly curl the forearm inward to force the biceps muscle into a strong contraction. Hold for two or three seconds, then return to starting position. Exhort students to "make a big muscle" and to "show me your muscles!" Four times; work up to eight. **A**

This exercise may also be performed one arm at a time, which may make it easier for some nursing home students to master it.

10) Back drops: Start with both arms extended upward, palms facing the front. Slowly bend your arms at the elbow, lowering hands towards the back of the shoulders. Try to touch the shoulders with the fingers. Then extend the forearms back up to starting position. Five times; work up to ten. **B,C**

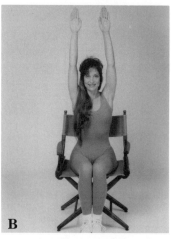

B

Remember that during this exercise your upper arm should never move. As your hands drop to the back, your elbows should remain pointing upward (instead of pointing to the front or to the sides). This exercise may also be performed using one arm at a time, which may make it easier for some nursing home students to master it.

11) The swim: Use your arms and shoulders to imitate a traditional-style swimming stroke. Ten times (five strokes per arm); work up to twenty. **D**

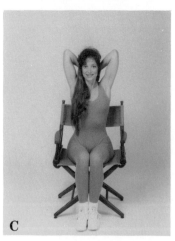

C

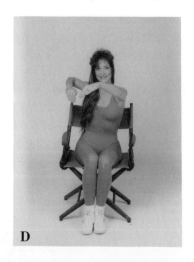

D

12) The breast stroke: Use your arms and shoulders to imitate the swimming breast stroke. Ten times; work up to fifteen. **A**

13) Alternate arm reaches high over head. Ten times (five per arm); work up to twenty. **B**

14) Alternate arm reaches forward at chest level. Ten times (five per arm); work up to twenty.

Wrists:

1) With fingers straight, move hands at a moderate speed up and down at the wrists. Make certain that students move hands only, not arms. Ten times (five up, five down); work up to twenty. **C,D**

2) Same as above, except alternate one hand up and then the other. Ten times (five up per hand); work up to twenty.

3) With hands and fingers straight, hold wrists side by side four to five inches apart. Without moving the arms, tilt your hands in sideways until fingertips touch. Then, on the same plane, tilt hands out sideways as

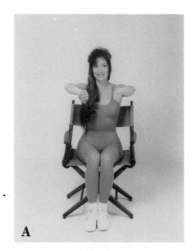

A

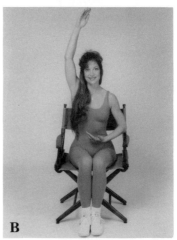

B

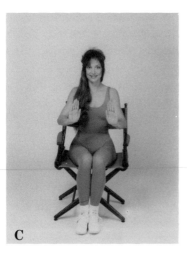

C

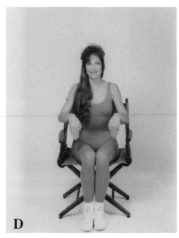

D

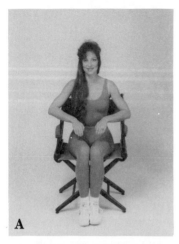

A

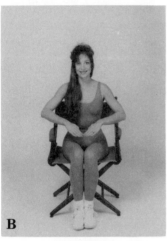

B

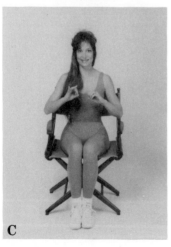

C

far as possible. Ten times (five in, five out); work up to twenty. **A,B**

Forearms/Hands/Fingers:

1) Rub hands together vigorously, creating friction and warmth. Thirty seconds to one minute.

2) Make loose fists with both hands. Release one finger at a time until all ten are stretched wide. Starting with the last finger released, fold one finger at a time back into the palm until you have two fists again. **C**

Nursing home students follow this exercise particularly well when you count forward to ten during the releases and backwards to one during the folds, which are in the opposite direction.

Abdomen:

1) Using the same principle as that in the abdominal exercise from Seniorcise Workout 1, contract and relax the abdomen at a moderate speed without holding. Five times; work up to fifteen.

This exercise should be taught only after students have mastered the abdominal exercise from Seniorcise Workout 1. Once they are proficient at controlling their muscles slowly, they will be able to alternately "flatten" and relax the abdomen at a quicker pace.

Waist:

1) Hold the arm of your chair with one hand. Lean and stretch downward towards the floor at the opposite side of the chair with the other arm. Return to an upright position. Five times; work up to ten. Repeat, using the other arm to stretch

downward towards the floor at the opposite side. Five times; work up to ten. **A**

You can make this exercise fun by saying, "Pretend that you've just dropped a one-hundred-dollar bill on the floor and you've got to try your best to reach down there and get it back!" Or, try variations such as trying to pick up the Hope Diamond or anything especially precious — let your students suggest valuable items worth a good stretch to retrieve. A limber student can be motivated to touch the floor if you capture his imagination with your presentation of this exercise.

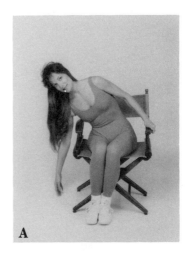

A

Buttocks:

1) Using the same principle as that in the buttocks exercise from Seniorcise Workout 1, contract and relax the buttocks muscles at a moderate speed without holding. Five times; work up to fifteen.

This exercise should be taught only after students have mastered the buttocks exercise from Seniorcise Workout 1. Once they are proficient at controlling their muscles slowly, they will be able to alternately squeeze and relax their buttocks at a quicker pace.

Lower Back:

1) Extend both legs straight to the front and hold. Stretching both arms towards your toes, slowly lean forward as far as feels natural and comfortable. Remain in this position for a few seconds (if comfortable). Then lower the legs and slowly raise back up to an upright position. Remain upright for five to ten seconds before repeating. Three times; work up to five. **B**

Upper Legs:

1) Repeat Exercise #4 from the Upper Legs section of Seniorcise Workout 1.

2) Repeat Exercise #5 from the Upper Legs section of Seniorcise Workout 1.

3) Repeat Exercise #6 from the Upper Legs section of Seniorcise Workout 1.

(The three exercises above are effective for both strength and flexibility while, at the same time, basic enough to be performed by most nursing home students. They are included in the upper legs sections of all Seniorcise workouts.)

4) Slowly lift and cross one leg over the

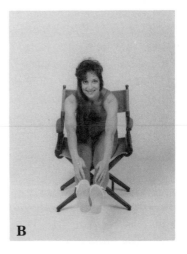

B

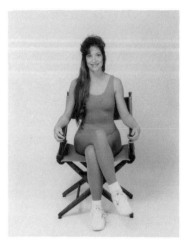

other. Remove it, and then cross the other leg over it. Ten times (five per leg); work up to twenty.

Some nursing home students will not be able to cross legs. Modify by asking them to try crossing at the ankles.

Ankles:

1) Start by extending both legs to the front high enough so that feet do not touch the floor. Then lift and lower the feet in an up-and-down motion at the ankles. Be careful to move only your feet, not your legs. Keep toes as relaxed as possible. Ten times (five up, five down); work up to twenty.

Lower Legs/Feet/Toes:

The following exercises should be performed barefooted or sock-footed.

1) Wriggle toes. At first, concentrate on moving your toes only (avoid up-and-down movement of feet at the ankles). Thirty seconds. Then permit feet to move up and down at the ankles as toes wriggle. Thirty seconds.

2) Curl toes under feet, then relax. Five times; work up to ten.

3) Spread toes as wide apart as possible, then relax. Five times; work up to ten.

Relaxation:

1) Close your eyes and stretch both arms high overhead. Hold for two or three seconds.

2) Slow pulls: With eyes still closed and arms still high, slowly imitate the motions of climbing a rope. Eight times (four slow pulls per arm).

3) Lower arms and relax for five to ten seconds.

4) Repeat Exercise #1 above.

5) Open eyes and slowly lower arms until palms rest on knees.

6) Rock forward and backwards gently as if you were in a rocking chair. Thirty seconds to one minute.

Senior Workout 3

Start your routine with the same Posture/Breathing exercises outlined in Seniorcise Workout 1. These basic exercises are the starters for all Seniorcise workouts.

Face:

1) Using small circular strokes, caress your face with your fingers. Be sure to include the eyebrows, the temples, and the lips. Do not apply pressure — just a soft, soothing touch. Thirty seconds to one minute.

2) Lift eyebrows as high as possible, then relax. Five times; work up to ten.

Neck:

1) Gently massage the back of your neck with your fingers. Do not massage the front of the neck, though, since that could inhibit blood flow. Thirty seconds to one minute.

2) Slowly turn the head in a pendulum motion from side to side, lowering chin toward the chest at the center and raising it slightly at the edges. This movement should be executed gently and conservatively. Six times (three toward each side).

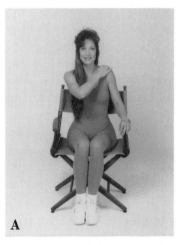

A

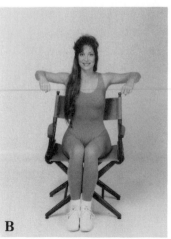

B

Upper Body (Shoulder Girdle/Upper Arms):

1) Place your right palm on your left shoulder. As you raise the shoulder, allow your right hand to "go along for the ride." Five times; work up to ten. Repeat, resting the left palm atop the right shoulder. Five times; work up to ten. **A**

2) Rowboats: Start with arms bent at shoulder level, elbows pointing towards the sides. Using a circular motion, imitate the action of rowing a boat. First, row forward. Ten times; work up to fifteen. Then without lowering the arms before changing directions, row backwards. Ten times; work up to fifteen. **B**

Nursing home students follow this exercise particularly well when you count forward during the forward rowing and backwards during the backward rowing. Or, they may enjoy singing, "Row, row, row your boat . . ." to accompany their movements. Rowing is my students' favorite calisthenic exercise, and we remember to include it in every workout.

3) Start by bending both hands into posi-

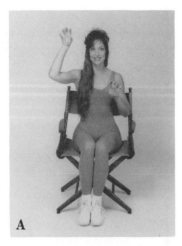

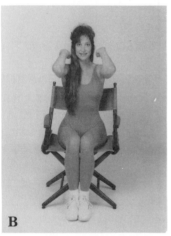

A

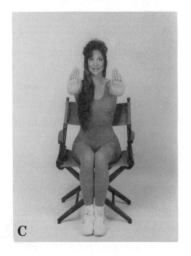

B

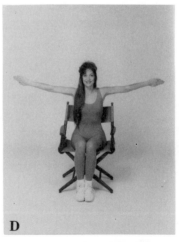

C

D

tions resembling cat claws, palms facing front. Then perform alternate arm reaches as if the cat were clawing on the door trying to get in your house. Ten times (five per arm); work up to twenty. **A**

4) Perform biceps curls as described in the Upper Body section of Seniorcise Workout 1, except fix elbows at shoulder level pointing towards the sides. Curl the forearms inward towards the top of your shoulders. Ten times; work up to fifteen.

5) Alternate biceps curls at sides: Same as above, except that as one forearm is lowered the other forearm is raised. Ten times (five curls per arm); work up to twenty.

6) Frontal extensions: Start with arms bent, elbows pointed toward the front at shoulder level, palms flexed facing upward. At a moderate speed, extend the forearms downward toward the front with the flexed palms facing forward. Return to starting position. Five times; work up to fifteen. **B,C**

7) Start with your arms extended out to sides at shoulder level, palms facing back. **D** Without moving upper arms, rotate forearms at a moderate speed down and in-

ward to the chest. Rotate back to starting position. Five times; work up to fifteen. **A**

8) Start with your arms bent at a ninety-degree angle at shoulder level, elbows pointing to the sides, palms facing front. Keeping the arms bent and the elbows level, rotate both inward at a moderate speed. When arms meet in front of the chest, try to touch them together (all the way from the elbows up through the fingertips). Rotate back to starting position. Five times; work up to fifteen. **B,C**

9) Extend your arms, palms down, to the sides at shoulder level. At a moderately fast speed, perform shallow up and down arm lifts. Fifteen to thirty seconds. Then without lowering or bending the arms before changing positions, move them to the front at chest level. Perform shallow arm lifts there. Fifteen to thirty seconds. Then relax arms to lap.

10) Same as above, except palms face upward. Fifteen to thirty seconds each way.

11) Extend both arms behind you, palms facing up. At a moderately fast speed, perform shallow up and down arm lifts. Fifteen to thirty seconds. **D**

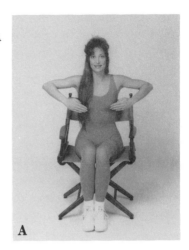

A

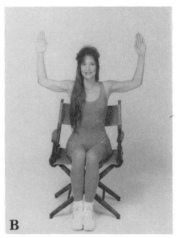

B

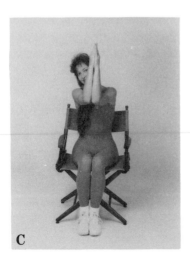

C

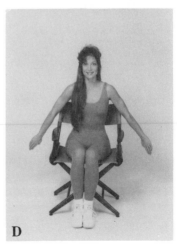

D

12) Rope climbing: With arms stretched high overhead, use a moderate speed to imitate the motions of climbing a rope. Your fingers should also be active during this exercise. Ten times (five pulls per arm); work up to twenty.

Wrists:

1) Repeat Exercises #1 and #2 from the Wrists section of Seniorcise Workout 1, except perform the circles with hands loosely fisted instead of with fingers straight.

2) Repeat Exercises #1 and #2 from the Wrists section of Seniorcise Workout 2, except perform the up and down movements with hands loosely fisted instead of with fingers straight.

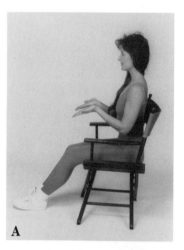

A

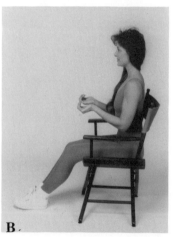

B.

Forearms/Hands/Fingers:

1) With palms facing upward, slowly curl first your fingers and then your hands inward over the inside of the wrists. Then, gradually unfold first your hands and then your fingers back out to starting position. Five times; work up to ten. **A,B,C**

2) Shake hands and fingers vigorously. Thirty seconds to one minute.

Abdomen:

1) Select either Exercise #1 from the Abdomen section of Seniorcise Workout 1 or Exercise #1 from the Abdomen section of Seniorcise Workout 2. When students are strong enough, you can include both exercises in the same workout.

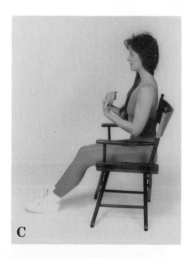

C

Waist:

1) Relax both arms downward to the sides (outside the arms of your chair). At moderately slow speed, lean first toward one side and then toward the other. Continue to alternate. Ten times (five to each side); work up to twenty. **A**

2) Extend both arms to the sides at shoulder level. At a moderately slow speed, reach as far to the side as possible with one arm and then as far as possible to the opposite side with the other arm. Continue alternating. Ten times (five to each side); work up to twenty. **B**

Buttocks:

1) Select either Exercise #1 from the Buttocks section of Seniorcise Workout 1 or Exercise #1 from the Buttocks section of Seniorcise Workout 2. When students are strong enough, you can include both exercises in the same workout.

Lower Back:

1) Extend the right leg straight out toward the front and hold. Extend the right arm straight out above it and hold. Slowly using both limbs, try to bring arm and leg together to touch. Return to the extended positions. Five times. Repeat, using left arm and leg. Five times. **C,D**

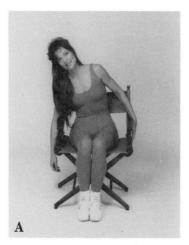

A

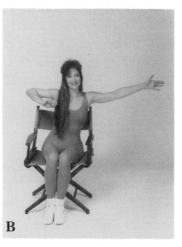

B

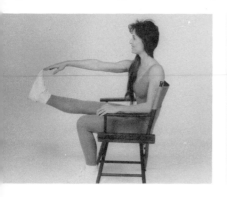

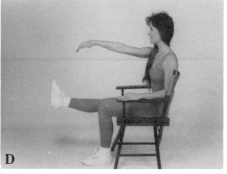

D

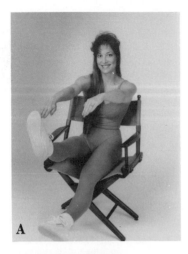

A

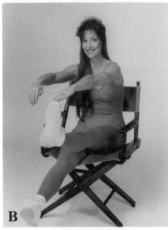

B

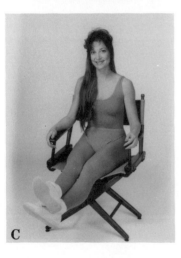

C

Be sure that the leg is moving upward to meet the arm as the arm simultaneously moves down towards the leg. Some nursing home students will tend to hold their legs stationary, depending on their arms to do all the work.

2) Same as above, except extend both legs and both arms. Without ever relaxing legs to floor or arms to lap, alternate bringing right limbs together and then left limbs together. Six times (three per side); work up to ten. **A,B**

Upper Legs:

1) Repeat Exercise #4 from the Upper Legs section of Seniorcise Workout 1.

2) Repeat Exercise #5 from the Upper Legs section of Seniorcise Workout 1.

3) Repeat Exercise #6 from the Upper Legs section of Seniorcise Workout 1.

(The three exercises above are included in the Upper Legs sections of all Seniorcise workouts.)

4) Extend your right leg to the front, heel resting on the floor. Cross the left leg over it at the ankle. Lift the right leg, allowing the left leg to "go along for the ride." Five times; work up to ten. Repeat with right leg crossed over left. Five times; work up to ten. **C**

5) With both feet lightly touching the floor, slide them back and forth vigorously. Thirty seconds to one minute.

Ankles:

1) Start by extending both legs to the front high enough so that feet do not touch the floor. Then bend the feet back and forth in a side to side motion at the ankles. Be careful to move only your feet, not your legs. Ten times (five each side); work up to twenty. **A,B**

Lower Legs/Feet/Toes:

1) Start with both feet flat on the floor. Raise your heels, shifting the weight of your feet onto your toes. Return heels to floor. Alternate. Ten times (five up, five down); work up to twenty. **C,D**

2) Shake feet vigorously. Fifteen to thirty seconds.

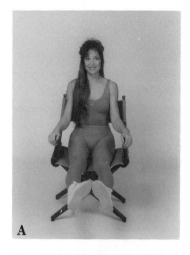

A

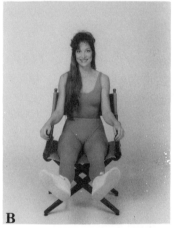

B

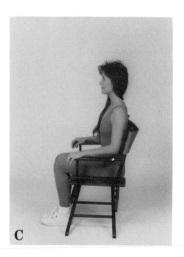

C

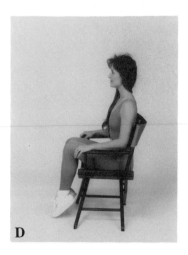

D

Relaxation:

1) Close your eyes and relax your hands in your lap. At a slow, soothing pace, sway from side to side with your shoulders. Thirty seconds.

2) With eyes still closed, recite to your students a poignant line of poetry or a brief quotation. Have them repeat it in unison. Instead of asking them to memorize the whole passage, just break it down into segments of a few words at a time. Check your public library for books of famous quotes and other inspirational literature. At the end of this chapter, you will find twenty-five of my students' favorite quotations to get you started.

In Closing

You can design your own Seniorcise routines by employing various combinations of the exercises described in the three illustrative workouts presented here. Be sure to include exercises from each body section listed in the workouts. Select exercises that move the joints in different ways and that work the main muscles located both in front and in back of your limbs and torso. When you practice an exercise listed under a specific body section, you will be able to feel which side of the body it is working. Let's take the arms for example. As a general rule, lifting/pulling movements work the biceps muscle while extension/pushing movements work the triceps. Therefore, biceps curls will exercise the front of your upper arm while pushups, back drops, and frontal extensions will exercise the back of it.

So, be creative. For variety's sake, do change exercise combinations from time to time. Always remember to include your students' favorite moves. And, have a terrific workout!

SUPPLEMENT

Below are twenty-five quotations suitable for use during the Relaxation section of Seniorcise Workout 3:

Where we love is home—home that our feet may leave, but not our hearts. — Oliver Wendell Holmes, Sr.

I'm not denyin' the women are foolish: God Almighty made 'em to match the men. — George Eliot

Could a greater miracle take place than for us to look through each other's eyes for an instant? — Henry David Thoreau

I see God in every human being. — Mother Teresa

Give the American people a good cause, and there's nothing they can't lick. — John Wayne

The way I see it, if you want the rainbow, you gotta put up with the rain. — Dolly Parton

A problem is a chance for you to do your best. — Duke Ellington

Experience is the name everyone gives to their mistakes.
— Oscar Wilde

The shell must break before the bird can fly. — Alfred, Lord Tennyson

Talk not of wasted affection. Affection never was wasted.
— Henry Wadsworth Longfellow

A fanatic is someone who can't change his mind and won't change the subject. — Winston Churchill

Wrinkles should merely indicate where smiles have been.
— Mark Twain

Truth is generally the best vindication against slander.
— Abraham Lincoln

No bird soars too high if he soars with his own wings.
— William Blake

What we wish, that we readily believe. — Demosthenes

The supreme happiness of life is the conviction that we are loved.
— Victor Hugo

To promise not to do a thing is the surest way in the world to make a body want to go and do that very thing. — Mark Twain

A sharp tongue is the only edge tool that grows keener with constant use. — Washington Irving

Nothing great was ever achieved without enthusiasm.
— Ralph Waldo Emerson

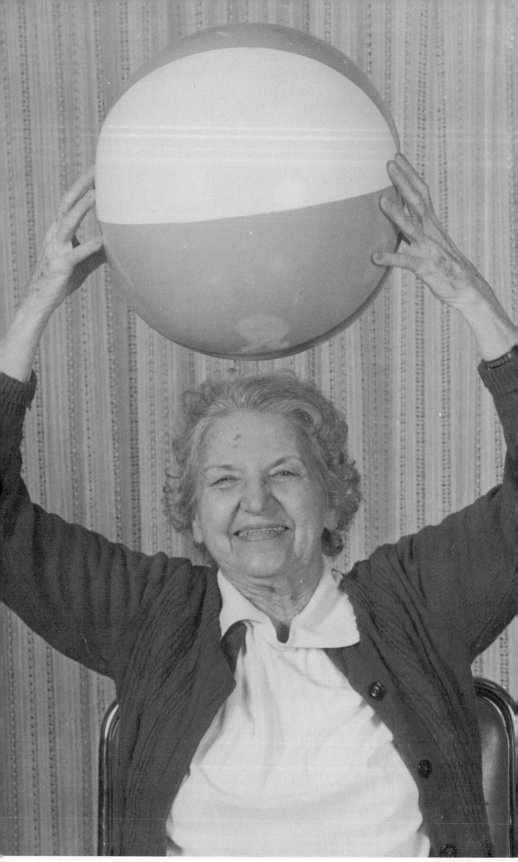

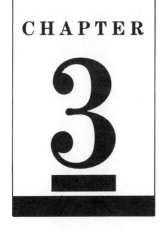

CHAPTER 3

The Phenomenal Urge to "Play Ball!"

For some mysterious reason, certain elderly students who don't respond to anything else will suddenly "come to life" when presented with a ball.

Gracie

Gracie, a ninety-year-old nursing home resident long confined to her wheelchair, was totally unresponsive during our first few meetings. She didn't speak or move at all. To me, she appeared to be out of touch with reality, lost in a quiet world that was all her own. The nurses presented her punctually for each meeting, and I thought it possible that perhaps Gracie gained some private benefit just from sitting amid the action and excitement of class. But I didn't think that she would ever be able to participate in fitness activities.

I was wrong. During the second week of the program, we held our first kickball game. To my surprise, Gracie not only took part — she never missed a kick!

Since that day, I've been increasingly more successful in getting Gracie to try a variety of exercises. But even on days when she seems unaware of our calisthenics, weight work, and mental stimulation games, she becomes instantly alert when I introduce the ball.

Irene, Gilbert and Katie

If the nursing home held an election to vote on the "most popular" lady in residence, Irene and Katie would probably tie. They both enjoy frequent visitors. They subscribe to newspapers and magazines. They take advantage of all the activities offered by the nursing home, including church services, music classes, art courses, and field trips. Gilbert is a favorite among his fellow residents and among the staff as well. He's a good listener and a well-informed conversationalist with a seemingly endless supply of fascinating

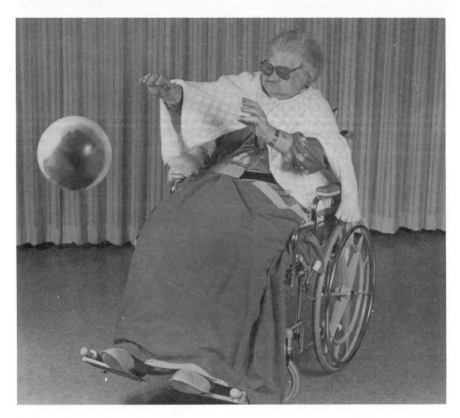

facts and anecdotes to share.

These residents sound like perfect candidates for group fitness class, don't they? Well, they are! They are also extremely discerning individuals with lots of other interests to follow (and plenty of other places to go) if fitness class bores them or offends them or fails to live up to their expectations.

Irene, Gilbert, and Katie have made it quite clear to me that kickball is their favorite fitness work. Irene even said, "I love to play ball! That's why I come to class." They do recognize the value of the other exercises, and their participation in the whole class is not only beneficial to them, but also helpful to me as the leader. So, you'd better believe, I *always* allot a little time for kickball, even when I've planned to conduct another sport or special activity during a given class.

In General

Conducting simple ball games can be a leader's most powerful tool for ensuring continued participation and for evoking maximal effort. In the heat of excitement generated by a lively kickball game, students will bend and stretch their trunks and move all four limbs about vigorously — without ever once thinking about the energy they are expending. They will burn off extra calories while sharpening eye-hand coordination and eye-foot coordination.

Keeping "your eye on the ball" and staying "on the ready" to return it necessitates prolonged mental attentiveness. And, best of all, ball games combine fitness with laughter and fun, a connection that you as the leader will certainly want your students to make.

The games included in this chapter do not require you to keep score, to split up into teams, or to single out winners. The group *is* a team which works together toward one easily comprehended goal, such as keeping the ball going in one direction or sustaining a long volley. In this simple, uncluttered context, you remain free to recognize and reward both group and individual accomplishments.

Naturally, some nursing home students will enjoy taking part in *competitive* sports which employ the use of balls. Instructions for two such games will be given in Chapter Four, "Sports and Special Activities."

What Type Ball Works Best?

As time goes by, you will probably accumulate a collection of balls having various textures, sizes, weights, and degrees of resiliency. Relatively speaking, balls are inexpensive fitness equipment and, therefore, easily approved for funding. This is good, because your students will literally wear balls out on a regular basis, and they will need to be replaced.

Only two kinds of balls are really necessary for nursing home fitness activities. The first type is small (four to five inches in diameter) and solid, though slightly porous. It should be made of soft, squeezable foamlike material. I use the popular Nerf ball, which is sold in most department, variety, and discount stores.

The second type is a large beachball (more than a foot in diameter). For safety purposes, you should use a very light *inflatable* type of beachball.

Always remember to select the brightest, most gayly colored balls that you can find for use in your nursing home fitness meetings.

More Safety Tips

Following the steps below will help to ensure that ball games run smoothly.

1) Set wheelchair brakes so that chairs do not roll during play.

2) Rotate wheelchair footrests up and out of the way.

3) The super-enthusiast may request that you remove the sides of his wheelchair (of which the footrests are a part). On most models, it is easy to slide them off and to slide them back on and secure them into place.

4) Make certain that lap robes do not drag on the floor or otherwise get in the way.

5) Angle chairs so that all students are able to achieve direct kicks. Make sure that amputees and stroke patients are aligned in positions advantageous to their useable limbs.

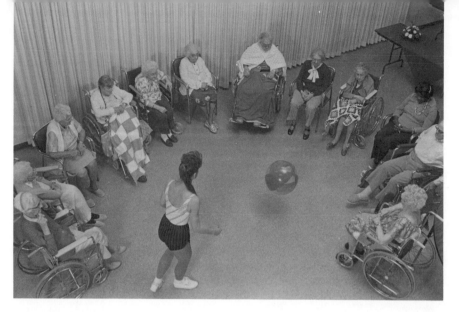

6) Position the strongest players across from each other. Do not permit a student whose attention tends to wander to sit in the line of fire of a spirited kicker. If a student is having trouble maintaining concentration, watch him closely. You may need to move him out of the active circle.

7) Infrequently, a player will doze off during play. Try rousing the sleepy student with some cheery conversation like: "Lisa, are you getting your beauty rest? We think you're already beautiful! Wouldn't you rather play ball with us?" If the player nods off again, guide her gently away from the field of play.

8) The student with a tender sore on his foot or elsewhere will not want to sit in the active circle during a ball game.

9) Students not seated in the active circle will enjoy watching from nearby, and you can make certain they get occasional opportunities to throw the ball either to you or into the circle.

Beachball Activities

1) **Seated Kickball:** The leader must be physically fit in order to conduct this game. The object of the game is to keep the ball going in the longest volleys possible; no specific pattern. The leader's duty towards this end will be to stay in the center of the circle, rerouting the ball as necessary. Whenever possible, redirect the ball without stopping it. *The leader must be extremely vigilant at intercepting any kick headed too fast towards an unprepared player.* In fact, you can prevent students from surprising each other with hard, fast kicks by giving logical instructions that stress safety, fun, and the goal of refining coordination skills. Make certain that all players get fair and frequent access to the ball. You will receive plenty of exercise running to retrieve the ball whenever it gets kicked outside the field of play.

But you can minimize this by placing empty chairs, either upright or on their sides, into any gaps that exist in the circle. When a student makes an exceptional play that keeps you from having to chase the ball, that is known as a *save*. Ambulatory students can take turns assisting you in some of the tasks described above.

Primarily, students will use their legs during kickball. But sometimes they will be called upon to slap or catch a ball that comes high or to the side. So teach them to *defend:* to protect their heads by using hands to knock the ball away.

You can make this exercise even more fun (and acknowledge good work at the same time) by providing play-by-play commentary during the game. A typical volley might run like this:

"I'll roll the ball to Anna for starters. Good return! Bill uses both feet to send it to Mary. Mary sends it on to Beth. Beth puts a spin on it! Now where's it going? Andy and Ella both get it, two-on-one! Saved by Alice! A good stretch for a line drive by John. You're all looking good. Perfect kick by Anna. All the way across the circle by Beth. Good, Alice! That's the way, Molly! Andy kicks a pop fly . . . and it's outta here!"

Then start all over, letting a different student be the first kicker.

2) **Pitch 'n' Pass:** Below are three workable variations for pitch 'n' pass.

    A. The leader goes around the circle to each student in turn. The leader tosses the ball to the student and then the student tosses the ball back to the leader.

    B. The ball goes around and around the circle in one direction with each student passing it on to the next. After a time, change directions.

    C. Students throw the ball around the circle in no specific pattern. They may throw to any player they wish including the leader, who stays in center circle to reroute and intercept as necessary.

3) **Combination Kickball:** Combine Exercise #1 above with Variation C of Exercise #2 above. The object of the game is to keep the ball going in the longest volleys possible, no specific pattern. A player may kick, slap, or catch and then throw the ball to any other player including the leader, who stays in center circle to reroute and intercept as necessary. Of all the activities I have ever supervised during nursing home fitness classes, this is the all-time favorite. Don't be surprised when games get loud and rowdy!

4) **Drop-Kick:** Go around the circle, letting each student in turn attempt to drop the ball with his hands and then kick it while it is still in midair. You can "play out" successful attempts that prove returnable. That is, keep it going in a volley for as long as possible.

5) **Dodgeball:** You're the target. See whether students can get the best of you, or whether you can elude their aim. Make sure that all players keep

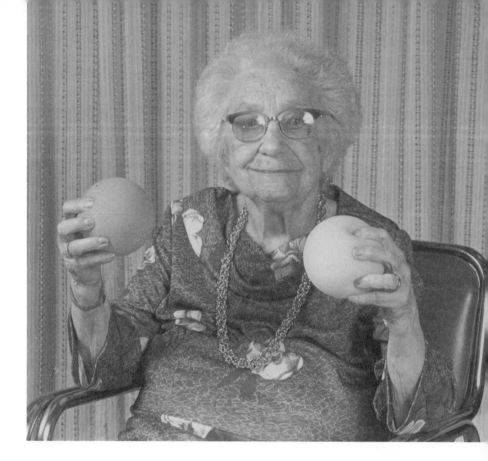

alert, ready to defend against tosses that miss you and head for them!

6) **"Last Call"**: At the close of beachball activities, some students will take you up on a "last call." One student may want one more chance to throw or catch the ball, or both. Another student may request one more kick. Another may request ten kicks in a row. Now is the time to encourage students to ask for and receive individual attention with the ball. Participants should also receive a resounding round of applause.

Nerf Ball Activities

1) Squeezes: If you have enough balls, pass one out to each student. Conduct a series of gripping exercises using first one hand and then the other to squeeze the ball. Include:

  A. Light, rapid squeezes. Ten times; work up to fifteen.
  B. Strong, slow squeezes. Five times; work up to ten.
  C. Tight squeezes held for a few seconds (if comfortable). Three times; work up to five.

2) If you only have one ball, send it around and around the circle. A given student squeezes it tight once with his right hand, passes it to his left hand,

squeezes once with his left, then passes it on to his neighbor on the left (who accepts it with his right hand). After a time, change directions.

If you have two balls, start the first going in one direction and the second heading in the opposite direction. Your students will get a chuckle out of coordinating things when the two balls meet at certain points during their rounds.

3) High tosses: Send the ball around and around the circle. Each student in turn attempts to throw the ball straight up as high as possible and to catch it. Then he passes it on to the next student. The leader should help students out by retrieving balls that get away from them. Ambulatory students may enjoy standing when they perform this exercise.

4) "Jacks": Send the ball around and around the circle. Each student in turn attempts to bounce the ball on the floor beside his chair and to catch it in mid-air on first bounce. Then he passes it on to the next student. The leader should help students out by retrieving balls that get away from them.

5) The waste basket toss: Carry a container around the circle, letting each student in turn attempt to "make a basket." Give each player several tries. Place the container on the floor in front of each student at a suitable distance, depending on his individual strength and skill. The container should be far enough away to represent a challenge, but close enough to ensure the possibility of successful aim. Adjust the distance as indicated after the student's first or second try.

As we will discuss in Chapter Four, this exercise can be easily modified to afford a competitive sports activity.

6) Repeat Pitch 'n' Pass (Exercise #2 — Variation A, B, or C — listed under Beachball Activities), except use a Nerf ball instead of a beachball.

7) Repeat Dodgeball (Exercise #5 listed under Beachball Activities), except use a Nerf ball instead of a beachball.

8) Repeat "Last Call" (Exercise #6 listed under Beachball Activities), except offer students the chance to repeat exercises that involve use of the Nerf ball.

In Closing

Ball games should be included in the Seniorcise meeting format during the segment set aside for a special activity or sports event. Additional Nerf ball activities will be discussed in Chapter Seven, "Working with the Elderly One-on-One."

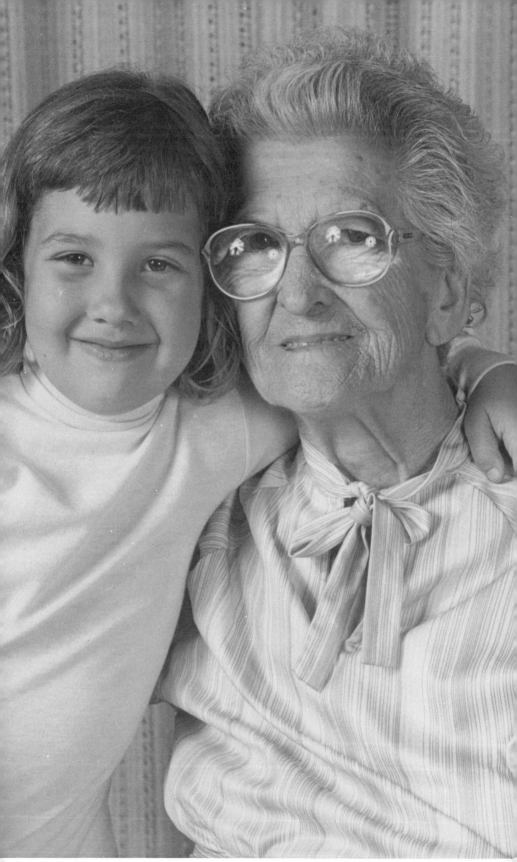

CHAPTER

4

Sports and Special Activities

An exciting modified sports event or special activity can "make" your elderly fitness student's day! Concerning sports contests, make certain that all participants have medical clearance to take part. Watch for stress signals as previously described in Chapter Two. In a nursing home environment, it is a simple matter to ensure that medical staff are in attendance or near at hand during sports activities. Remember that intense rivalry will serve only to frustrate participants and take the fun out of a game. Instead, create a mood of athletic camaraderie in which participating ranks right at the top with winning. Under these condittions, your students will be able to relax and enjoy all the fun.

How to Use This Chapter

The Seniorcise fitness class format suggests that every meeting be divided into three separate segments: 1) a supervised exercise workout, 2) a special activity or sports event, and 3) an intellectual game designed to promote mental fitness. This book is designed to provide you with a variety of activities for each separate segment from which you can easily select one activity to use at every meeting. So, in addition to the ball activities described in Chapter Three, these following activities are recommended for use during the segment set aside for a special activity or sports event.

Icebreakers

Icebreakers are especially useful during the beginning of a new program but can also be fun for a change any time. When icebreakers are used, you will usually want to hold the special activity segment at the beginning of your meeting.

1) Go around the group circle, letting each student in turn answer the question: What is your full name? Most students will be able to answer this

question and will enjoy pausing to discuss the origins of unusual names or to tease friends who admit they always hated their middle names.

2) Same as above. Question: Where are you from? Or, where did you grow up? Some students may be surprised to discover that they were practically neighbors long ago and didn't know it. Pause to discuss the pros and cons of growing up in the places students mention.

3) Same as above. Question: How many brothers and sisters did you grow up with in your family? It is quite likely that some students will report growing up in very large families. Pause to discuss whether they had especially close or favorite siblings, how they divided the family chores, and what their family gatherings were like at Thanksgiving and Christmas.

4) Same as above. Question: What is your favorite color? The gregarious student may be able to elaborate as to *why* he favors a certain color. Pause occasionally to ask a given student if he has many clothes of his favorite color or if he ever decorated a room in his favorite color.

5) Same as above.

    A. Think of your own question.

    B. Ask your students to suggest a question. If no student responds with an idea, urge the group to use their imaginations: "Just think! What one question would you like to put to everybody in this room?" If that fails, try to prompt a response by using humor and by offering examples: "OK, now's your chance to get nosey! Don't you want to know who in here has ever been to see an X-rated movie? Or how about, What is your worst habit?" Don't be surprised if students suggest your own examples back to you. Do go around the circle answering all questions contemplated during the activity.

6) As described in Chapter One, walk around the group circle shaking hands and greeting students by name. Then have students turn and shake hands with their neighbors on either side.

7) Same as above, except teach students a nontraditional handshake such as the "Peace" handshake (which was popular during the 1960's) or "Gimme Five" (which involves swapping light smacks on the palms).

Simple Simon Says

Traditionally, Simple Simon Says calls for one player to issue a series of commands to a group of fellow players. Any command that starts with the phrase *Simple Simon Says* should be followed, but any command not preceded by the phrase should be ignored. When a player complies with a command in error, he is eliminated from the round. The last remaining player wins the round and the right to give commands during the next round. Our game is played just like conventional Simple Simon Says with the following modifications:

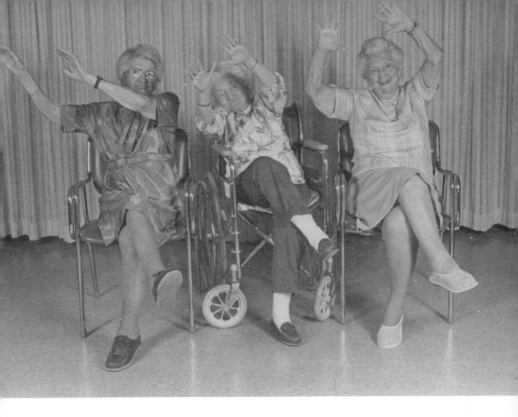

1) I think you will find that many students do not want to *be* Simple Simon. Therefore, you do not need to single out winners. Instead, the leader can play against the group as a team. If you do not mention Simon and the group obeys directions anyway, say, "Gotcha!" If not, say, "I didn't fool you!" Or there's, "I got a few of you on that one." And, to recognize individual excellence, "Ida's the only one who didn't fall for it."

2) Played in this manner, the game can go on indefinitely — as long as your students are enjoying themselves.

3) Played in this manner, you can let any student who wants to be Simple Simon take over as the leader for as long as he likes. Encourage students to try it.

4) Use exercises as the tasks that Simple Simon decrees. See the Upper Body and Legs sections of the Seniorcise workouts in Chapter Two for ideas.

Wheelchair Dance

Wheelchair dancing is a pleasurable activity as long as you keep the songs short (about three minutes) and the routines repetitive and simple. If your choreography is too elaborate, some nursing home students won't be able to follow it, and others won't cooperate because it is "too much work." The guidelines below will help you to develop practical wheelchair dance routines.

1) All movements should be performed while seated. This way, wheelchair-bound and ambulatory students will be able to do identical routines together.

2) Routines which require students to roll forwards and backwards will exhaust some students and will be resisted by others who anticipate exhaustion. In a nursing home setting, it is usually advisable to let students dance in place.

3) Use simple movements such as: nodding, swaying from side to side, clapping hands, snapping fingers, punching, reaching, slapping knees, (seated) kicking, and toe tapping.

4) Members enjoy using tunes that they recognize such as "Alexander's Ragtime Band" or "Tea for Two."

5) Physical motions should match the music. Before planning a routine, listen carefully to the song you have chosen. Ask yourself which movements will lend themselves naturally to its particular pace and rhythm. Try out different moves until you have identified several that are complementary.

6) Select no more than four or five motions to use in one number.

7) Identify the main divisions of the song. For example, a typical song might be structured like this:

1. Introductory musical chords	6. Brief musical solo
2. Verse I	7. Verse III
3. Chorus	8. Chorus
4. Verse II	9. Final musical chords
5. Chorus	

8) Designate a movement for each segment of the song. Let's take the song in Guideline #7 above. If your group needs a very simple routine, you might choreograph that number like this:

1. During all three musical sections — sway from side to side.
2. During all three verses — tap toes.
3. During all three choruses — clap hands.

If your group can follow a more complex routine, the same number might work like this:

1. During all three musical sections — sway from side to side.
2. During Verse I — tap toes.
3. During Verse II — reach overhead with arms.
4. During Verse III — snap fingers.
5. During all three choruses — clap hands.

9) If your group would enjoy a routine more complex than either of the two outlined in Guideline #8 above, try including more than one movement in each verse or more than one movement in the chorus. Also, try alternating movements, for example snap/clap/snap/clap or reach up/reach out/reach up/reach out.

Shows and Entertainment

Your community is probably blessed with many talented persons willing to come into your nursing home and perform for the residents free of charge. Try to schedule live entertainment that will inspire participation while helping to keep members up-to-date on current events.

My group responds well to aerobic dance shows performed by members from my "outside" programs. Instead of just watching passively, they join right along with the whoops and stretches.

They also especially enjoyed a demonstration by my troupe of preteen breakdancers. After the show, the boys helped them to master some breakdance arm movements, including the "King Tut" and the "roller coaster."

Check with local exercise clubs, dance studios, and karate academies about the possibility of engaging volunteer performers. Explain that since the spectators belong to a fitness group, you are interested in entertainment that will to some degree involve them as participants.

If your nursing home owns a large-screen television and a VCR, you can play a fitness-related program for your students. One day I showed my students a thirty-minute exercise video that I had made. They thoroughly enjoyed seeing their leader "on TV" and they were able to perform many of the exercises on the tape. But you don't have to go out and make a video in order to conduct this activity! Check local video shops for tapes that demonstrate gentle exercise or tapes that deal with health matters pertinent to elderly students. Video rentals are inexpensive, and chances are that your nursing home already belongs to a video rental club.

Volunteer Assistants

Nursing home residents always enjoy seeing a new face. So whenever you can, bring a friend or an acquaintance along to class to assist with the sports and games.

The faces that delight nursing home residents most of all are those that belong to children. Children make terrific volunteer assistants. They have lots of energy for chasing runaway balls during kickball games. They're good at setting up bowling pins. And they make fine dodgeball targets, as well.

If several children are helping out with a dodgeball game, have the children take turns going into the circle. When one child gets hit, the next gets to

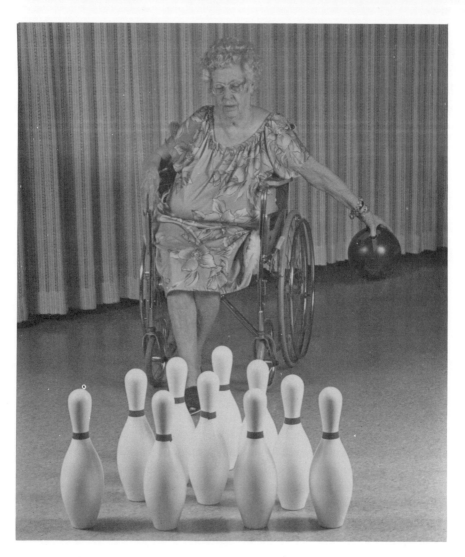

go in. Assign a set order of entry to prevent the children from having misunderstandings among themselves.

During blackboard games, some children enjoy doing the writing. Others like to take part in the game right along with the elderly class members. If a child is providing all the answers before members have a chance to speak up, just tell him that he's too smart for the rest of you. Then have him raise his hand before answering in order to give others time to respond, too.

Bowling

Your nursing home may be able to purchase a bowling set that includes ten light plastic pins and a ball with several holes of various sizes to accommodate both large and small hands. But when it comes to playing, the conventional rules for scoring can get complicated. Nursing home students enjoy bowling competitively when the rules are easy to understand and follow.

To start a game, list all the players' names on a blackboard. Each player will receive two consecutive turns. If he knocks down all ten pins on his first turn, he gets ten points. Write the score beside his name. Since he still has one more turn, set up the pins again. If he knocks down all ten pins, he gets ten more points for a total of twenty (if he only knocks down four, his total is fourteen). Say that the next player knocks down eight pins on his first turn. Give him eight points, and then have him use his second turn to try for the two leftover pins (for a maximum possible total of ten points).

If two or more players tie for top score, they can continue competing against each other until the tie is broken. If you wish, you can have the finalists roll the ball a longer distance during the tie-breaker rounds.

Pins should be set up in a triangular configuration including four rows of one, two, three, and four pins. Marking each pin's position on the floor with a small piece of masking tape makes set-up quick and easy.

Masking tape can also be used to mark the lines on the floor behind which a bowler must stay during his turns. You will need two lines, one for players using wheelchairs (five to ten feet away from the pins) and one for standing players (ten to twenty feet away from the pins). The first time your group bowls together you'll be able to determine exactly where to place lines in order to set up the fairest possible match.

Competitive Waste Basket Toss

Go around the group circle to each player in turn. You will need only one container. After a player takes his turn, move it in front of the next player. Using a tape measure, place the container 36 inches away from the front leg of the player's chair.

List all the players' names on a blackboard. Each player will receive two consecutive turns to try to "make a basket" with the Nerf ball. He may score zero, one, or two points. Record his score on the board beside his name.

Two or more players will probably tie for top score. They can continue competing against each other until the tie is broken. If you wish, you can have the finalists throw the ball a longer distance during each tie-breaker round (from 36 inches to 48, then 60, then 72, etc.).

Variation: At the start of a game say, "We're going to go around three times before we tally the scores, so everyone will get two shots at three different times during the game." This works especially well for small groups. Break ties in the same manner as described above.

Special note: The origins of this game's name go back to the austere beginnings of the Seniorcise program! But these days we use a lovely woven wicker basket, which tends to enhance the activity.

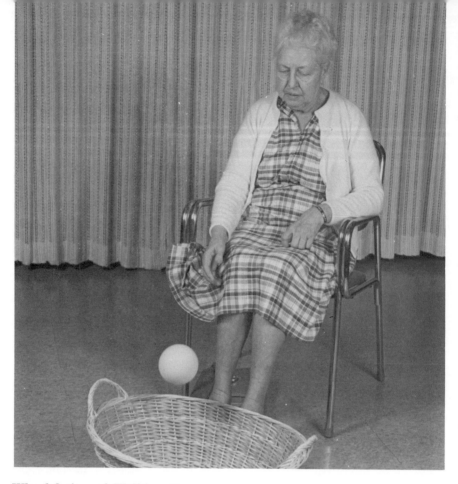

Wheelchair and Walking Races

During the first wheelchair race I ever held, one of my students insisted that she could roll faster backwards than forwards. I was skeptical, but she proved her point by coming in second place! I learned my lesson, and now I encourage students to do things *their* way.

When you hold a race, keep your track straight and short (twenty to twenty-five feet). Place masking tape on the floor to mark start and finish lines clearly. Just match two or three contenders at a time. The winners from round one then race against each other. Continue eliminating until you have a winner.

Have someone at the finish line to help wheelchair students get slowed down after they cross.

You can make this activity even more fun by promoting lots of good-natured rooting and enthusiastic cheering. Students who are unable to participate will thoroughly enjoy watching the races as will staff members who are free to attend.

Use the same rules along with the same start and finish lines to conduct

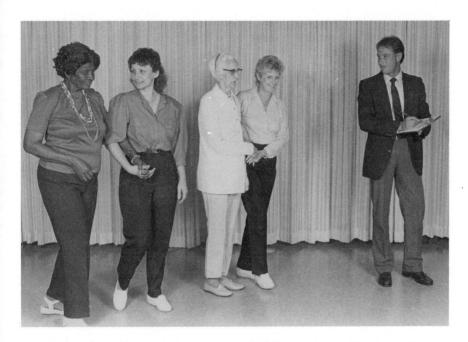

a walking race for your ambulatory students. You and your volunteer assistants can serve as escorts, providing each student with a steady arm and seeing that he sets a comfortable, non-stressful pace.

Avoid matching ambulatory students against students who use wheelchairs. Instead, have a champion "walker" and a champion "roller." Each will reign supreme and will defend his title the next time you hold a race.

Obstacle Races

Use a straight track twenty-five feet long. Place masking tape on the floor to mark start and finish lines. Place three plastic bowling pins in the middle of each contestant's pathway: the first at five feet, the second at ten feet, and the third at fifteen feet. (Empty bleach bottles make fine substitutes for bowling pins. If you don't have a bowling set, ask the nursing home laundry to donate used bottles.) At twenty feet, place a Nerf ball (or a beachball) on a chair *beside* each contestant's pathway. Place one basket (or other large container) on the middle of the finish line.

Since contestants will need plenty of room during this activity, you should match only two contenders at a time (it also requires less equipment, provides equal access to the basket, and permits you space to get in and remove pins as they are kicked over). The racer must kick over the first pin before proceeding past it to the next. He must kick over the second pin before proceeding to the third. He must kick over the third pin before

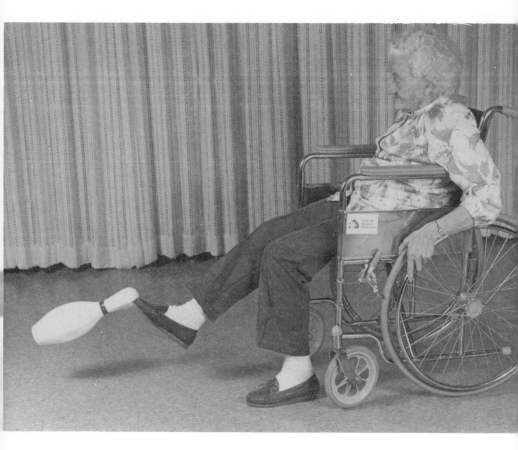

proceeding to the ball. He must then pick up the ball, carry it to the finish line, place it in the basket, and cross the finish line himself. Winners from round one then race against each other. Continue eliminating until you have a winner.

As in the regular wheelchair race, have someone at the finish line to help wheelchair participants get slowed down after they cross.

As in the regular walking race, assign an escort to each walking participant.

Avoid matching ambulatory students against students who use wheelchairs. Instead, hold two separate competitions and have a champion "walker" and a champion "roller."

The Seniorcise Multi-Sport Tournament

Set aside an entire meeting period for this extra-special event. Using the rules and guidelines in this chapter, let students compete in the following sports: a bowling match, a competitive waste basket toss, a wheelchair race, a walking race, a wheelchair obstacle race, and a walking obstacle race.

Announce the tournament ahead of time in your nursing home newsletter. Be sure to invite family members, staff members, and the local press as well. Since you will probably be too busy to visit or grant interviews, why not prepare a program for your guests? It should include students' names, a schedule of tournament events, and some general information about the other fitness activities that the group performs regularly.

Organize everything possible in advance, so that the tournament will run smoothly. For example, try to sign students up for the events they wish to enter before the day of the tournament. Do, however, get last-minute enthusiasts into the games if they change their minds!

Make a list of all the equipment to be used and make sure that it is handy before you start. Also, prepare the necessary start and finish lines in advance. And, don't forget the camera! In fact, if the nursing home owns a video camera, students will enjoy viewing a tape of the event later.

Line up nursing home staff members and assistants to take responsibility for the following jobs:

- to greet guests and distribute programs,
- to serve refreshments,
- to take pictures,
- to film or tape the event,
- to escort walking race participants,
- to help wheelchair racers get slowed down after crossing the finish line,
- to call winners at the finish line,
- to set bowling pins,
- to keep the scoreboard,
- to award ribbons, prizes, and certificates.

Reward all the participants with certificates and white ribbons for entering. Award first, second, and third place event winners ribbons colored to denote their rankings. If one student wins more single events than anyone else, award him an ornate ribbon and/or a grand prize and declare him the Champion Seniorcise Athlete. Some nursing homes will be able to provide prizes such as powder, lotion, guest soaps, stuffed animals, or even cash.

Note: In most nursing home fitness groups the ladies and gentlemen will be able to compete fairly together on an equal basis. But all students need the chance to practice these games during regular class meetings before participating in a tournament. Doing so also gives the leader an opportunity to time the games. Eliminating down to second and third place in each contest is time-consuming. You may prefer to determine first place winners only. Timing events in advance prepares you to make sound plans.

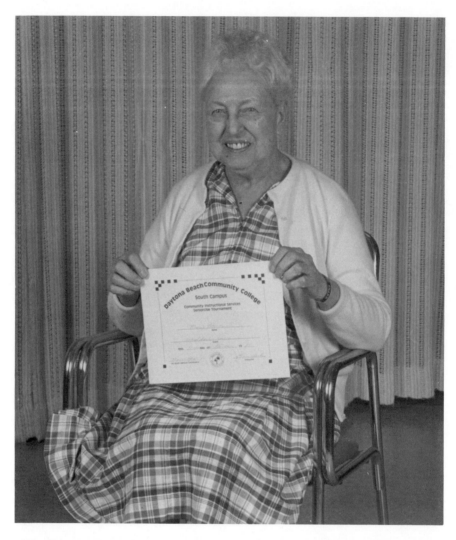

Find out if the nursing home can furnish refreshments for the residents and the guests. Involve the students themselves in tasks such as preparing the scoreboard and greeting new arrivals. Get a good night's rest before the big day. In other words, do everything possible to ensure that your Seniorcise Multi-Sport Tournament is an entertaining, memorable event.

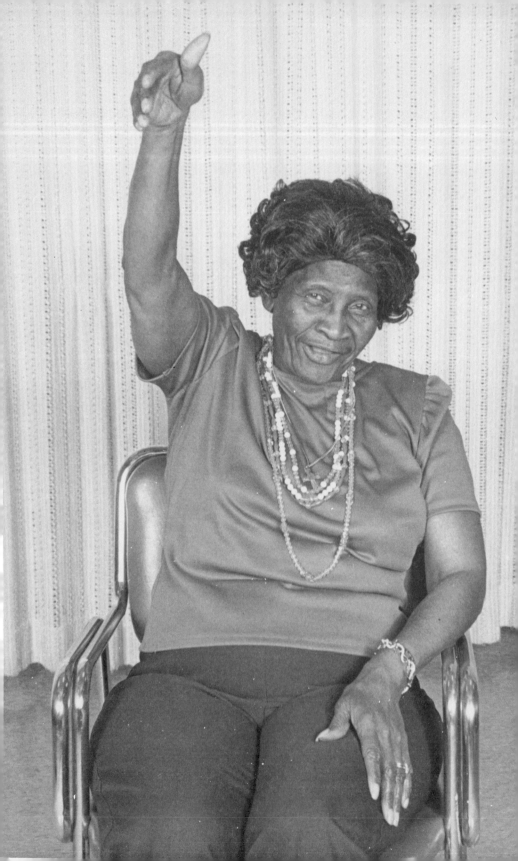

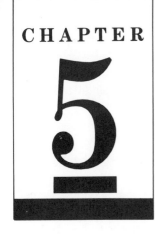

CHAPTER 5

Fun Games for Mental Fitness

Current research suggests that the mental backsliding commonly associated with old age can, in many cases, be prevented through the use of simple games designed to exercise the mind.

Most elderly persons are not senile. They may, however, encounter fewer and fewer situations that demand prolonged concentration or that necessitate quick intellectual response. Without sufficient stimulation, they may appear to undergo some degree of mental disintegration. Or, they may begin to feel that they're just not as "sharp" as they used to be.

Every Seniorcise meeting will include one cognitive activity which should be conducted during the segment set aside for mental fitness. The leader must see to it that games are never childish or demeaning, but are, instead, appropriate for adults. With that in mind, I am providing instructions only for the activities that have become favorites with my students. A special emphasis has been placed on relating simple activities — games in which cognitively-impaired adults can participate successfully, thereby deriving mental stimulation. Students who require greater intellectual challenges will favor the more demanding games, for example Major Cities or list games with topics (such as dog breeds) that involve a limited number of correct answers.

All of the intellectual games described in this chapter are designed to promote mental activity. My students call this component of the program their "brain exercise." They have a lot of fun *stretching* their imaginations and giving their brain cells a *workout!*

Note: *Exercise for the brain* is a figurative phrase. Since the brain is not actually a muscle, we cannot make it stronger by flexing it in a literal sense. We can, however, employ other methods to activate it.

I have described the Seniorcise mental fitness program to the major American researchers presently conducting investigations into the effects of aging on intellectual abilities. The consensus among the researchers is that these Seniorcise games are extremely worthwhile. There is evidence that continued intellectual/social activity can help to maintain cognitive functions, increase sensory awareness, and preserve social skills. Seniorcise mental fitness games are designed to play that role.

Making the Most of Attention Spans

If you simply say, "We're going to play a game now," without further explanation to your nursing home fitness students, you may get responses such as these: "Games are for children"; "I don't feel like playing a game"; or "I'm tired. I think I'll go to my room."

What's going wrong here? The leader is failing to motivate his students.

Introduce games for mental fitness by explaining exactly what they are. They are *intellectual* games. They are *adult-oriented*. You might say, "Now that we've exercised the rest of our bodies, we'd better work on our brains, too." Students should be told that mental exercises represent an integral part of their balanced, overall fitness plan. They should come to expect a sit-down workout, a sport or special activity, and a mental exercise at every meeting. They need to know that any given drill makes sense, that they are going to get something out of it over and above gratifying a teacher who wants to see them play a game. If, at the same time, their leader successfully presents the task as a "labor of fun," he will lay the kind of groundwork that encourages each student to apply himself with a positive attitude.

Once the activity is under way, help the nursing home fitness student to control his train of thought by making frequent references to the major theme or subject of the game. If the game generates discussion or debate, students can get sidetracked. When concentration begins to flag, unobtrusively guide the conversation back around to the topic at hand.

Cueing

When your students tackle a cognitive game, you can help them by offering well-placed suggestions aimed at jogging memory and provoking additional thought.

At the beginning of a game, students may have trouble channelling their thoughts along the specific lines of the exercise. Later on, they may reach a point (or points) at which they are just plain stumped.

One way to prompt a student is to repeat the object of the game. For example: "OK, Margaret. We're trying to list all the different types of animals that we can think of. So far we have cats, dogs, and horses. What other kind of animal can you call to mind?"

Providing a fresh example can also be effective. For example: "I know another one! Hamsters!" Better still, try using an example that suggests a whole new train of thought for students to pursue. For example: "How about the hippopotamus?" (to open up the category of zoo/jungle animals).

Put a picture into the student's mind. For example: "Think of a barnyard. What kinds of animals would we find there?" Or: "Picture all the animals that must have been on Noah's ark."

Descriptions, clues, and hints make good cues. For example: "Which animal loves cheese but hates cats?" Or: "Which animal carries a hump on his back and thrives in the desert?"

Catchwords or well-known sayings work well, too. For example: "If someone is very crafty, we might call him a sly *what*?" Or: "Hey diddle diddle, the cat and the fiddle. *What* jumped over the moon?"

When other methods fail, you can supply the first sound or syllable of a solution. For example: "No one remembers which animal has black and white stripes? Zzzzee . . ."

Along with the activity instructions provided in this chapter, I have included some supplemental cues that proved particularly effective for my nursing home students. Just remember to exercise your own little gray cells while your students are exercising theirs, and you will be able to come up with lots of cues to help make their intellectual efforts successful.

Let's take a look at the games themselves.

Complete the Quote

Provide students with the first few words of a famous saying or phrase, and have them try to supply the rest of it. Let students speak out separately or in unison as soon as they know an answer. After the game, ask them to try to think of other well-known sayings and quotations.

Below are enough samples for two complete games.

Game One

1. You can lead a horse to water — but you can't make him drink.
2. It takes one — to know one.
3. The pot is calling — the kettle black.
4. An apple a day — keeps the doctor away.
5. Out of sight — out of mind.
6. Don't look a gift horse — in the mouth.
7. A penny saved — is a penny earned.
8. You can't take it — with you.
9. Pretty is as — pretty does.
10. Absence makes the heart — grow fonder.
11. Can't, never — could.
12. You can't teach an old dog — new tricks.
13. Neither a lender nor — borrower be.
14. Don't upset the — apple cart.

15. Don't rock the — boat.
16. A rolling stone — gathers no moss.
17. If you can't say anything nice — don't say anything at all.
18. When the going gets tough — the tough get going.
19. Water, water everywhere — but nary a drop to drink.
20. Experience is the best — teacher.

Game Two

1. It takes money — to make money.
2. Nothing ventured — nothing gained.
3. Diamonds are a girl's — best friend.
4. What's good for the goose — is good for the gander.
5. Easy come — easy go.
6. All's fair in — love and war.
7. You'll catch more flies with honey than with — vinegar.
8. A man is known by — the company he keeps.
9. What goes up — must come down.
10. One bad apple doesn't — spoil the bunch.
11. Curiosity killed — the cat.
12. You can't keep a good man — down.
13. You're as old as — you feel.
14. Honesty is the best — policy.
15. Lie down with dogs — get up with fleas.
16. A man's home — is his castle.
17. Too many cooks — spoiled the broth.
18. Silence is — golden.
19. There's no place — like home.
20. A stitch in time — saves nine.

Grab Bag

This activity helps to coordinate sense of touch with mental perception. Prepare by filling a large bag with a variety of small articles, such as a golf ball, a bar of soap, a glove, a coaster, or a coin. Go around the group circle, letting each student in turn reach into the bag. First, he grasps and handles one item. Then, without looking into the bag, he tries to identify what he's holding. After announcing his conclusion, he pulls the item out to display before the group.

Needless to say, this game provides plenty of occasion for applause and laughter. Be careful not to include items that are sharp or otherwise dangerous. Powder puffs, plastic spatulas, lipstick tubes, potholders, tennis balls, and hair brushes all make good choices. Just look around your kitchen and bath for safe and interesting objects, and change the contents of your bag periodically.

Major Cities

This game is the most popular mental fitness activity of all among my class members.

Having prepared in advance a list from an atlas, name a principal city of the United States. Have your students try to guess which state it is in. Let students call out separately or in unison whenever they think they know an answer. Cue students with hints such as: "This is a very old city located in a southern state"; "This city is its state's capital"; "This city is in the Buckeye State"; and "This city is in our largest state."

My group turned out to be so knowledgeable and well travelled that they graduated to naming the countries in which principal cities of the world are located. When conducting this variation, cue students with hints such as: "This city is located on the South American continent"; "This city is located in the country that produced Napoleon"; "The people who live in this city might play bagpipes"; and, "This city is in the country that once carried out a famous inquisition."

Below are enough samples for four complete city/state games and two complete city/country games.

Game One

1. Nome — Alaska
2. Memphis — Tennessee
3. Milwaukee — Wisconsin
4. Providence — Rhode Island
5. Oshkosh — Wisconsin
6. Abilene — Texas
7. Akron — Ohio
8. Bakersfield — California
9. Baltimore — Maryland
10. Greensboro — North Carolina
11. Laredo — Texas
12. Las Vegas — Nevada
13. Louisville — Kentucky
14. Key West — Florida
15. Ithaca — New York
16. Iowa City — Iowa
17. Huntingdon — Pennsylvania
18. Huntington — Indiana, New York, and West Virginia
19. Cadillac — Michigan
20. Dallas — Texas
21. Daytona Beach — Florida
22. Gary — Indiana
23. Syracuse — New York
24. San Francisco — California
25. Raleigh — North Carolina
26. Sharon — Pennsylvania
27. Roanoke — Virginia
28. Fresno — California
29. Charlotte — North Carolina
30. San Jose — California
31. St. Paul — Minnesota
32. Birmingham — Alabama
33. Ann Arbor — Michigan
34. Atlanta — Georgia
35. Butte — Montana
36. Little Rock — Arkansas
37. Chicago — Illinois
38. Cheyenne — Wyoming
39. Catskill — New York
40. Walla Walla — Washington
41. Topeka — Kansas
42. Erie — Pennsylvania
43. Tulsa — Oklahoma
44. Tampa — Florida
45. San Diego — California

Game Two

1. Seattle — Washington
2. Baton Rouge — Louisiana
3. Boise — Idaho
4. Jersey City — New Jersey
5. Kalamazoo — Michigan
6. Houston — Texas
7. Laramie — Wyoming
8. Bethlehem — Pennsylvania
9. Annapolis — Maryland
10. Hannibal — Missouri
11. Bridgeport — Connecticut
12. Asheville — North Carolina
13. Phoenix — Arizona
14. New Orleans — Louisiana
15. Santa Rosa — California
16. Santa Fe — New Mexico
17. Reading — Pennsylvania
18. Hackensack — New Jersey
19. Sioux Falls — South Dakota
20. Long Beach — California
21. Spartanburg — South Carolina
22. Astoria — Oregon
23. Boston — Massachusetts
24. Oakland — California
25. Macon — Georgia
26. Pueblo — Colorado
27. New Brunswick — New Jersey
28. Chattanooga — Tennessee
29. Detroit — Michigan
30. Fort Worth — Texas
31. Durham — North Carolina
32. Tacoma — Washington
33. Orlando — Florida
34. Wheeling — West Virginia
35. Tucson — Arizona
36. Anniston — Alabama
37. Niagara Falls — New York
38. New Bedford — Massachusetts
39. Peoria — Illinois
40. Corpus Christi — Texas
41. Santa Barbara — California
42. Saginaw — Michigan
43. Reno — Nevada
44. Savannah — Georgia
45. New York City — New York

Game Three

1. Miami — Florida
2. Philadelphia — Pennsylvania
3. Oklahoma City — Oklahoma
4. Selma — Alabama
5. San Antonio — Texas
6. Albuquerque — New Mexico
7. Great Falls — Montana
8. Schenectady — New York
9. Atlantic City — New Jersey
10. Indianapolis — Indiana
11. El Paso — Texas
12. Shreveport — Louisiana
13. Boulder — Colorado
14. Montgomery — Alabama
15. Buffalo — New York
16. Hoboken — New Jersey
17. Sioux City — Iowa
18. Amarillo — Texas
19. Freeport — Illinois
20. South Bend — Indiana
21. Cedar Rapids — Iowa
22. Nebraska City — Nebraska
23. Sacramento — California
24. Toledo — Ohio
25. Spokane — Washington
26. Augusta — Georgia
27. Tombstone — Arizona
28. Utica — New York
29. Santa Cruz — California
30. Pensacola — Florida
31. Minneapolis — Minnesota
32. Arlington — Massachusetts
33. Vancouver — Washington
34. Des Moines — Iowa
35. San Bernardino — California
36. Huntsville — Alabama
37. Waco — Texas
38. Sumter — South Carolina
39. Colorado Springs — Colorado
40. Fredericksburg — Virginia
41. Yazoo City — Mississippi
42. Salt Lake City — Utah
43. Galveston — Texas
44. Denver — Colorado
45. Nashville — Tennessee

Game Four

1. Cincinnati — Ohio
2. Fort Wayne — Indiana
3. Wichita — Kansas
4. Amsterdam — New York
5. Tuscaloosa — Alabama
6. Carson City — Nevada
7. Marblehead — Massachusetts
8. Allentown — Pennsylvania
9. Yonkers — New York
10. Terre Haute — Indiana
11. Newport News — Virginia
12. Bismarck — North Dakota
13. Andover — Massachusetts
14. St. Augustine — Florida
15. Fayetteville — North Carolina and Arkansas
16. Mechanicsville — New York
17. Knoxville — Tennessee and Pennsylvania
18. Beaver Falls — Pennsylvania
19. Santa Monica — California
20. Talladega — Alabama
21. White Plains — New York
22. Waycross — Georgia
23. Pasadena — California
24. Dubuque — Iowa
25. Pittsburgh — Pennsylvania and Kansas
26. Biloxi — Mississippi
27. Shenandoah — Pennsylvania
28. Princeton — New Jersey and Indiana
29. Bedford — Indiana
30. Mason City — Iowa
31. Cleveland — Ohio and Tennessee
32. Duluth — Minnesota
33. Tonawanda — New York
34. Dayton — Ohio and Kentucky
35. Trenton — New Jersey and Missouri
36. Suffolk — Virginia
37. Flint — Michigan
38. Englewood — New Jersey and Florida
39. Albany — New York and Georgia
40. Berkeley — California and Virginia
41. Charlottesville — Virginia
42. Mobile — Alabama
43. Tallahassee — Florida
44. St. Louis — Missouri
45. Los Angeles — California

Game Five

1. Hong Kong — China
2. Berlin — Germany (West and East)
3. Montreal — Canada
4. Florence — Italy
5. Liverpool — England
6. Madrid — Spain
7. Marseilles — France
8. Limerick — Ireland
9. Copenhagen — Denmark
10. Hiroshima — Japan
11. Guadalajara — Mexico
12. Munich — West Germany
13. Cairo — Egypt
14. Belfast — Northern Ireland
15. Cordova — Spain and Argentina
16. Ottawa — Canada
17. Calcutta — India
18. Havana — Cuba
19. Cuzco — Peru
20. Glasgow — Scotland
21. Cannes — France
22. Dresden — East Germany
23. Dublin — Ireland
24. Chungking — China
25. Hamburg — West Germany
26. Dunkirk — France
27. Genoa — Italy
28. Granada — Spain and Nicaragua
29. Gloucester — England and United States (Massachusetts)
30. Hanoi — Vietnam
31. Athens — Greece
32. Moscow — Russia
33. Leeds — England
34. Lima — Peru
35. Oxford — England
36. Palermo — Italy
37. Melbourne — Australia
38. Edinburgh — Scotland
39. Geneva — Switzerland
40. Manchester — England
41. Naples — Italy
42. Frankfurt — West Germany
43. Delhi — India
44. Panama — Panama
45. Paris — France

Game Six

1. London — England
2. Nagasaki — Japan
3. Cambridge — England (and U.S., Massachusetts)
4. Antwerp — Belgium
5. Barcelona — Spain
6. Budapest — Hungary
7. Bombay — India
8. Monterrey — Mexico (and U.S., California, spelled Monterey)
9. Luxemburg — Luxemburg
10. Algiers — Algeria
11. Bordeaux — France
12. Calgary — Canada
13. Canterbury — England
14. La Mans — France
15. Nassau — The Bahamas
16. Bern — Switzerland
17. Dusseldorf — West Germany
18. Lancaster — England
19. Amsterdam — Netherlands
20. Brussels — Belgium
21. Brisbane — Australia
22. Lisbon — Portugal
23. Nuremberg — West Germany
24. Milan — Italy
25. Exeter — England
26. Nice — France
27. Managua — Nicaragua
28. Buenos Aires — Argentina
29. Oslo — Norway
30. Bonn — West Germany
31. Dunedin — New Zealand (and U.S., Florida)
32. Caracas — Venezuela
33. Bogota — Columbia
34. Derby — England
35. Cork — Ireland
36. Nottingham — England
37. Bhopal — India
38. Cologne — West Germany
39. Avignon — France
40. Dundee — Scotland
41. Lyon — France
42. Quebec City — Canada
43. Dover — England
44. Mexico City — Mexico
45. Washington, D.C. — United States.

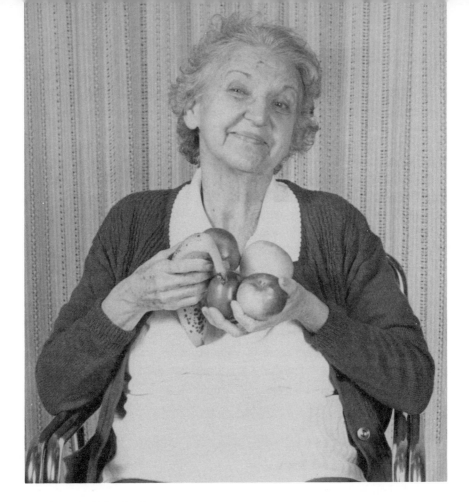

How Many Calories?

This activity calls for the use of logic. Students use the process of elimination to narrow down the range of possible answers until they arrive at the correct one. The game gets easier as they go, because as more and more foods are added they gain more points of reference for comparison. Meanwhile, everyone gets a nutrition lesson, too.

To start, list several widely divergent types of food on a blackboard. Using large, clear handwriting, place each food's calorie count beside it. Good examples include:

One piece of blueberry pie — 250 calories
One slice of pot roast — 300 calories
One apple — 70 calories
One head of lettuce — 50 calories.

Explain that you will write the name of a specific type of food on the board. The object of the game is for the students to guess how many calories it contains. Before they begin playing, give them some general guidelines to help them arrive at the correct solutions. You might say, for instance: "We all know that eating a lot of certain foods will put fat on a person, while eating other, more natural foods will help him to stay slim. The foods that cause us to add fat are generally higher in calories than those that don't. That piece of blueberry pie contains so many calories because it is packed with sugar. And the pot roast is high in calories because it contains a lot of fat. So, those are the two things to look for while you're playing this game. Foods that are loaded with sugar and fat are going to have the most calories. Natural foods, on the other hand, will contain fewer calories. Notice that the fresh apple only has seventy calories. And a *whole* head of lettuce only has fifty. So, with that in mind, let's see if you can guess the number of calories contained in some other foods."

Round the calorie counts off to numbers divisible by five. Let students call out their guesses separately or in unison. Keep them on the right track by using cues such as: "Good guess. You're getting warm"; "That's close. It's just a little higher"; and, "Remember that this dish is prepared with a lot of sugar, so it's going to have quite a few calories." Always end the game with a question that most of your students will be able to answer readily, so that they will finish on a triumphant note.

Below are enough samples for four complete games.

Game One

	Calories
1. 1 tangerine	40
2. 1 c. apple juice	120
3. 1 c. baked beans prepared with pork and molasses	325
4. 1 T. jam, jelly or preserves	55
5. 1 tomato	35
6. 1 slice corned beef	270
7. 1 stalk celery	5
8. 1 piece caramel candy	40
9. 1 spear broccoli	10
10. 1 slice white bread	70
11. 1 piece chocolate fudge	65
12. 1 c. Brussels sprouts	45
13. 1 slice pumpernickel bread	65
14. 1 Fig Newton	55
15. 1 spear asparagus	5
16. 1 piece watermelon	115
17. 1 slice rye bread	65
18. 1 whole cantaloupe	120

19. 1 piece chocolate cream candy 50
20. 1 piece pumpkin pie 230
21. 1 c. orange juice 110
22. 1 slice rib roast 240
23. 1 c. grapefruit juice 95
24. 1 chocolate mint patty 40
25. 1 piece apple pie 300

Game Two

1. 1 orange... 70
2. 1 pear.. 100
3. 1 T. sugar 50
4. 1 whole egg 80
5. 2/3 c. chocolate or
   vanilla ice cream 200
6. 1 c. shredded cabbage 15
7. 1 T. honey 65
8. 1 roasted chicken leg 100
9. 1 c. cream of mushroom soup 110
10. 1 T. margarine 100
11. 1 c. cream of green pea soup.............................. 110
12. 1 T. mayonnaise 100
13. 1 roasted chicken thigh 140
14. 1 T. molasses 50
15. 1 c. chicken noodle soup 55
16. 1 c. sliced yellow squash 30
17. 1 c. chicken vegetable soup................................ 60
18. 1 c. strawberries 55
19. 1 T. maple syrup.. 60
20. 1 piece lemon meringue pie 270
21. 1 T. peanut butter.. 95
22. 1 persimmon 75
23. 1 c. sliced pineapple 75
24. 1 nectarine 50
25. 1 piece cherry pie 300

Game Three

1. 1 carrot 20
2. 1 slice poundcake... 140
3. 1 piece French bread 110
4. 1 frozen chicken pot pie................................... 450
5. 1 slice plain cake
   with no icing... 200

6. 1 banana 85
7. 1 piece Italian bread....................................... 110
8. 1 frozen beef pot pie 450
9. 1 slice chocolate cake
    with chocolate icing 440
10. 1 grapefruit... 90
11. 1 ear corn 70
12. 1 ounce American process cheese 105
13. 1 onion 40
14. 1 c. cherries 80
15. 1 frozen turkey pot pie 450
16. 1 ounce cheddar cheese 105
17. 1 c. whole milk... 150
18. 1 c. skim milk.. 90
19. 1 ounce Swiss cheese 120
20. 1 c. blackberries.. 85
21. 1 oz. blue cheese 105
22. 1 c. buttermilk 90
23. 1 c. evaporated milk 345
24. 1 piece mincemeat pie 300
25. 1 c. blueberries 85

Game Four

1. 1 cucumber 30
2. 1 doughnut 125
3. 1 lemon 20
4. 2 oz. whiskey 160
5. 1 artichoke 30
6. 1 corn muffin 150
7. 1 c. diced yellow turnips 50
8. 1 c. raspberries 70
9. 1 cupcake with icing 185
10. 1 c. spinach.. 40
11. 2 oz. rum.. 160
12. 1 brownie.. 120
13. 1 green pepper... 15
14. 1 biscuit 130
15. 1 c. carbonated soft drink 100
16. 1 c. green beans 30
17. 1 beer... 100
18. 1 slice bologna 80
19. 1 radish 1

20. 1 fig 30
21. 1 slice bacon 50
22. 1 c. cooked egg noodles 200
23. 1 plum 25
24. 1 c. cooked rice 200
25. 1 peach 35

The Amen Game

This activity combines mental exercise with physical exercise.

Ask the group a series of questions. Any time that a student can answer *yes* to a specific question, he should wave both arms vigorously overhead and call out: "AMEN!" (Or, you can use a different catch phrase such as "YES, INDEED!"). If his answer is *no*, he remains still and quiet. At the end of the game, ask students if they can think of other related questions to ask.

Below are enough samples for ten complete games.

Game One

1. Are you at least twenty years old?
2. Are you at least thirty years old?
3. Are you at least forty years old?
4. Are you at least fifty years old?
5. Are you at least sixty years old?
6. Are you at least seventy years old?
7. Are you at least eighty years old?
8. Are you at least ninety years old?
9. Are you at least one hundred years old?
10. Were you born in January?
11. Were you born in February?
12. Were you born in March?
13. Were you born in April?
14. Were you born in May?
15. Were you born in June?
16. Were you born in July?
17. Were you born in August?
18. Were you born in September?
19. Were you born in October?
20. Were you born in November?
21. Were you born in December?
22. Are your eyes blue?
23. Are your eyes brown?
24. Are your eyes green?

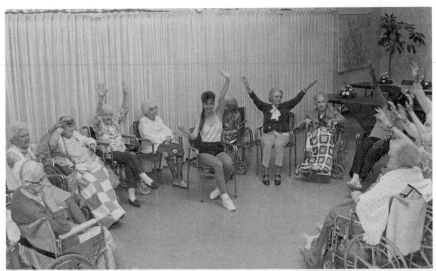

25. Are your eyes gray?
26. Did you eat breakfast this morning?
27. Have you had lunch yet?
28. Are you going to eat dinner tonight?
29. Have you heard a radio today?
30. Have you watched any TV today?

Game Two

Question: Have you ever heard this song?
1. America the Beautiful
2. My Country 'tis of Thee
3. The Star-Spangled Banner
4. The Battle Hymn of the Republic
5. Dixie
6. Old Man River
7. It Ain't Necessarily So
8. Summertime
9. The Sound of Music
10. Climb Every Mountain
11. Oklahoma
12. Somewhere Over the Rainbow
13. Camptown Races
14. Smoke Gets in Your Eyes
15. Boogie Woogie Bugler Boy
16. In the Mood
17. Row Row Row Your Boat
18. Twinkle Twinkle Little Star
19. My Way
20. The Green Leaves of Summer
21. The Impossible Dream
22. Moon River
23. Hello, Dolly
24. Cabaret
25. Born Free
26. Way Down Upon the Swanee River

Game Three
Question: Have you ever heard of this organization or of this type of club?

1. A book club
2. A record club
3. A bridge club
4. A garden club
5. A ski club
6. A boat club
7. A gun club
8. A hunting club
9. A golf club
10. A country club
11. An exercise club
12. A union
13. A college fraternity
14. A college sorority
15. An honor society
16. A historical society
17. The Chamber of Commerce
18. The Republican party
19. The Democratic party
20. A USO club
21. The VFW
22. The Procrastinators' Club
23. The Optimists' Club
24. The Boy Scouts
25. The Girl Scouts
26. The Campfire Girls
27. The AAA Auto Club
28. The AARP (for retired persons)
29. The American Legion
30. The Knights of Columbus
31. The Masons
32. The Jaycees
33. The Eagles
34. The Elks
35. The Lions
36. The Moose
37. The Rotary

Game Four
Question: Have you ever heard of this famous animal?

1. Fury
2. Flicka
3. Traveler
4. Lassie
5. Rin Tin Tin
6. Old Yeller
7. Goofy
8. Snoopy
9. Huckleberry Hound
10. Fred Basset
11. Marmaduke
12. Morris the Cat
13. Thomasina
14. Topcat
15. Garfield
16. Bill the Cat
17. The Pink Panther
18. Mighty Mouse
19. Mickey Mouse
20. Atom Ant
21. Donald Duck
22. Daffy Duck
23. Bugs Bunny
24. Roadrunner

Game Five

Question: Have you ever heard of this type of music or musical group?

1. Jazz
2. Swing
3. Blues
4. Country
5. Western
6. Folk
7. Bluegrass
8. Dixieland
9. Gospel
10. Chamber
11. Rock 'n' roll
12. Bubblegum
13. Pop
14. Soul
15. Easy listening
16. Minstrel singers
17. A string quartet
18. A barbershop quartet
19. A marching band
20. A jug band
21. A boys' choir
22. The Mormon Tabernacle Choir

Game Six

Question: Have you ever heard of this magazine?

1. Better Homes and Gardens
2. Business Week
3. Cosmopolitan
4. Ebony
5. Family Circle
6. Field & Stream
7. Forbes
8. Fortune
9. Harper's Bazaar
10. House Beautiful
11. Ladies' Home Journal
12. Life
13. Look
14. McCalls'
15. Money
16. Newsweek
17. Outdoor Life
18. People
19. Playboy
20. Prevention
21. Reader's Digest
22. Redbook
23. Southern Living
24. Time
25. True Romance
26. Vogue
27. Woman's Day
28. Yankee

Game Seven

Question: Have you ever heard of this store? (Add stores that are popular in your region.)

1. Ace Hardware
2. A&P
3. Belks
4. Bi-Lo
5. Bloomingdale's
6. Eagles
7. Eckerds
8. Family Dollar Store
9. Fayva Shoe Store
10. Gimbel's
11. Hallmark Shop
12. K-Mart
13. Lerner's
14. Loehmann's
15. Lord and Taylor
16. Macy's
17. Majik Market
18. Neiman Marcus
19. Pantry Pride
20. JC Penney
21. Pic'n'Pay
22. Pier I
23. Piggly Wiggly
24. Roses
25. Sears
26. Seven Eleven
27. Spencer Gifts
28. Toys 'R' Us
29. Waldenbooks
30. Walgreen's
31. Western Auto
32. Winn Dixie
33. World Bazaar

Game Eight

Question: Have you ever heard of this poet or writer?

1. William Blake
2. Elizabeth Barrett Browning
3. Pearl Buck
4. Lord Byron
5. Lewis Carroll
6. Chaucer
7. Agatha Christie
8. Stephen Crane
9. Samuel Coleridge
10. Charles Dickens
11. Emily Dickinson
12. T.S. Eliot
13. Ralph Waldo Emerson
14. William Faulkner
15. Rachel Field
16. F. Scott Fitzgerald
17. Robert Frost
18. Robert Graves
19. Nathaniel Hawthorne
20. Ernest Hemingway
21. Homer
22. Victor Hugo
23. John Irving
24. James Joyce
25. Franz Kafka
26. John Keats
27. Stephen King
28. Rudyard Kipling
29. D.H. Lawrence
30. Sinclair Lewis

Game Nine
Question: Have you ever heard of this poet or writer?

1. Henry Wadsworth Longfellow
2. Walter de la Mare
3. Christopher Marlow
4. Herman Melville
5. Edna St. Vincent Millay
6. Margaret Mitchell
7. Edgar Allen Poe
8. Ellery Queen
9. Carl Sandburg
10. William Shakespeare
11. Percy Bysshe Shelley
12. John Steinbeck
13. Robert Louis Stevenson
14. Jonathan Swift
15. Alfred, Lord Tennyson
16. Dylan Thomas
17. Henry David Thoreau
18. J.R.R. Tolkien
19. Leo Tolstoi
20. Mark Twain
21. John Updike
22. Leon Uris
23. Kurt Vonnegut
24. H.G. Wells
25. Thornton Wilder
26. Walt Whitman
27. Williams Wordsworth

Game Ten
Question: Have you ever heard of this musical instrument?

1. Accordian
2. Bagpipe
3. Banjo
4. Bass
5. Bassoon
6. Bells
7. Cello
8. Clarinet
9. Cymbal
10. Drum
11. Fiddle
12. Fife
13. Flute
14. French horn
15. Guitar
16. Harp
17. Harpsichord
18. Horn
19. Kazoo
20. Kettle drum
21. Lyre
22. Mandolin
23. Oboe
24. Organ
25. Piano
26. Pipe
27. Saxophone
28. Sitar
29. Spoons
30. Triangle
31. Trombone
32. Trumpet
33. Tuba
34. Ukulele
35. Violin
36. Washboard
37. Xylophone

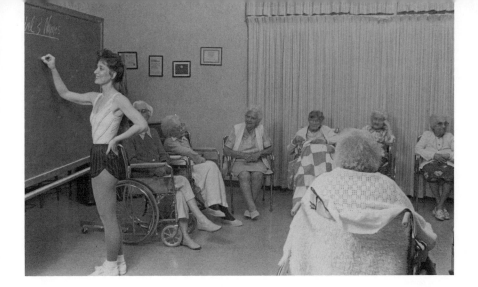

The List Game

Agree on a general topic, and have the students try to think of as many items as possible which can be associated with it. Write each item on a blackboard in order to prevent redundancy. Let students call out their ideas separately or in unison.

I have by no means attempted to list here all the possible answers for any given game. You and your students will think of many original solutions that I haven't included. But enough answers have been listed to provide the leader with plenty of solutions towards which to aim students, through the use of cues, when they reach impasses during the game. You will be able to devise your own cues, too, but I have occasionally included cues that I found particularly helpful in guiding students towards certain answers.

Below are enough samples for ten complete games.

Game One

Try to list as many animals and birds as you can think of.

House pets:
1. Cat
2. Dog
3. Hamster
4. Gerbil
5. Guinea pig

Farm animals:
6. Mouse
7. Rat
8. Horse
9. Pony
10. Mule
11. Donkey
12. Cow
13. Ox
14. Goat
15. Sheep

Woodland creatures:

16. Bobcat
17. Mountain lion
18. Panther
19. Cougar
20. Wolf
21. Coyote
22. Jackal
23. Hyena (Cue: the laughing *what?*)
24. Fox
25. Bear
26. Buffalo
27. Deer
28. Elk
29. Wild boar
30. Groundhog (Cue: If he sees his shadow, winter will continue)
31. Mole
32. Prairie dog
33. Chipmunk
34. Squirrel
35. Rabbit
36. Hare (Cue: From *Alice in Wonderland,* the mad hatter and the March *what?*)
37. Raccoon
38. Opossum (Cue: Plays dead)
39. Porcupine
40. Skunk
41. Muskrat
42. Otter
43. Beaver (Cue: Known for building dams)

Jungle animals:

44. Lion
45. Tiger
46. Gorilla
47. Ape
48. Monkey
49. Orangutan
50. Chimpanzee
51. Mandrill (Cue: A monkey whose face is colored in brilliant shades of red and blue)
52. Zebra
53. Gazelle
54. Wildebeest (Cue: Also known as the gnu)
55. Giraffe
56. Mongoose (Cue: Famed for skill at killing snakes)
57. Elephant
58. Hippopotamus
59. Rhinoceros

Foreign animals:

60. Camel (Cue: Egypt, hump on back)
61. Kangaroo (Cue: Australia, pocket on his stomach
62. Koala bear (Cue: Australia, cuddly like a teddy bear)
63. Llama (Cue: Peru, a South American camel)
64. Lemming (Cue: Norway, they migrate en masse and jump into the sea)

Fowl: (Note — You can list birds as a totally separate game, depending on how much time you have spent on the animals.)

65. Canary
66. Parakeet
67. Parrot
68. Chicken
69. Turkey (Cue: Thanksgiving dinner)
70. Duck
71. Goose
72. Pigeon
73. Quail
74. Partridge (Cue: *What* in a pear tree?)
75. Dove (Cue: Represents peace)
76. Pheasant (Cue: *what* under glass?)
77. Owl (Cue: Wise old *what?*)
78. Peacock (Cue: Colorful fan of tailfeathers)
79. Eagle (Cue: The national bird)
80. Buzzard (Cue: Thrives on carrion)
81. Vulture
82. Crow (Cue: A scare-*what?*)
83. Ostrich (Cue: Buries head in the sand)
84. Pelican (Cue: Stores fish in pouch under beak)
85. Crane
86. Flamingo (Cue: Pink)
87. Swan (Cue: What the Ugly Duckling became)
88. Redbird
89. Bluebird
90. Blackbird
91. Bluejay
92. Mockingbird
93. Hummingbird
94. Magpie
95. Nightingale (Cue: The famous nurse, Florence *what?*)
96. Thrush
97. Wren
98. Finch

Game Two

Try to think of as many names as possible to give to a baby boy. (Cue: What were your fathers, brothers, and male friends named?)

1. Abraham (Cue: Lincoln)
2. Allen
3. Amos
4. Andrew
5. Ben
6. Bill
7. Bob
8. Brad
9. Bryan
10. Carl
11. Charles (Cue: Lady Diana and Prince *what?*)
12. Chester
13. Christopher (Cue: Columbus)
14. Clint (Cue: Eastwood)
15. Clyde (Cue: Bonnie and *who?*)
16. Dan
17. Dean
18. Dennis
19. Don
20. Ed (Cue: The talking horse)
21. Emil
22. Ernest (Cue: Hemingway)
23. Eugene
24. Frank
25. Fred
26. George
27. Gerald (Cue: Ford)
28. Glen (Cue: Miller)
29. Gordon
30. Hal
31. Hank (Cue: Williams)
32. Harold
33. Henry
34. Jack
35. Jake
36. James
37. Jeff
38. Jim
39. John
40. Julian
41. Kenneth
42. Larry
43. Lawrence (Cue: Olivier)
44. Lenny (Cue: Bruce)
45. Luke
46. Mack (Cue: *What* the Knife?)
47. Mark
48. Martin
49. Michael
50. Mike
51. Neil
52. Olin
53. Oliver (Cue: Charles Dickens' book, *Who* Twist?)
54. Oscar (Cue: The award)
55. Patrick (Cue: the saint; March 17th)
56. Paul
57. Peter
58. Quincy (Cue: President John *Who* Adams?)
59. Rick
60. Robert
61. Ronald (Cue: Reagan)
62. Sam
63. Samuel
64. Scott (Cue: F. *Who* Fitzgerald?)
65. Simon
66. Ted
67. Tim
68. Todd
69. Wayne
70. William

Game Three

Try to list all fifty states. (Cue: Give clues that help to describe the states such as: the "Longhorn State" for Texas; the hula dance and grass skirts for Hawaii; the "Sunshine State" for Florida; the river after which it is named for Mississippi; and the potato for Idaho. Or, try geographic hints such as: "There's one more southern state and it's located right under Virginia.")

1. Alabama	35. Ohio
2. Alaska	36. Oklahoma
3. Arizona	37. Oregon
4. Arkansas	38. Pennsylvania
5. California	39. Rhode Island
6. Colorado	40. South Carolina
7. Connecticut	41. South Dakota
8. Delaware	42. Tennessee
9. Florida	43. Texas
10. Georgia	44. Utah
11. Hawaii	45. Vermont
12. Idaho	46. Virginia
13. Illinois	47. Washington
14. Indiana	48. West Virginia
15. Iowa	49. Wisconsin
16. Kansas	50. Wyoming
17. Kentucky	
18. Louisiana	
19. Maine	
20. Maryland	
21. Massachusetts	
22. Michigan	
23. Minnesota	
24. Mississippi	
25. Missouri	
26. Montana	
27. Nebraska	
28. Nevada	
29. New Hampshire	
30. New Jersey	
31. New Mexico	
32. New York	
33. North Carolina	
34. North Dakota	

Game Four

Try to list as many things as possible that you would be likely to find at a school.

1. Classrooms
2. Desks
3. Tables
4. Blackboards
5. Chalk
6. Erasers
7. Notebooks
8. Textbooks
9. Rulers
10. Slide rules
11. Dunce caps
12. Paddles
13. Apples for the teacher
14. Tests and examinations
15. Report cards
16. Science lab
17. Microscopes
18. Dissecting tools
19. Bunsen burners
20. Library
21. Card catalog
22. Computers
23. Film projectors
24. Television sets
25. Auditorium
26. Stage
27. Stage curtains
28. Lectern
29. Band room
30. Piano
31. Musical instruments
32. Band uniforms
33. Cafeteria
34. Teachers' lounge
35. Offices
36. Fire alarms
37. Lockers
38. School buses
39. Gym
40. Basketball court
41. Tennis court
42. Baseball field
43. Football stadium
44. Sports equipment
45. Teachers
46. Principal
47. Guidance counselor
48. Secretaries
49. School nurse
50. Dietitian
51. Cafeteria staff
52. Janitors
53. Students
54. Parents

Game Five

Try to list all the television shows you can remember.

1. Father Knows Best
2. My Three Sons
3. The Dick Van Dyke Show
4. Leave it to Beaver
5. Dennis the Menace
6. I Love Lucy
7. I Married Joan
8. The Life of Riley
9. The Honeymooners
10. The Real McCoys
11. Car 54 — Where Are You?
12. Amos and Andy
13. My Mother the Car
14. Mr. Ed
15. My Favorite Martian
16. My Little Margie
17. The Dobie Gillis Show
18. The Adams Family
19. The Munsters
20. Superman
21. Batman
22. F-Troop
23. Green Acres
24. Hogan's Heroes
25. The Beverly Hillbillies
26. Gilligan's Island
27. The Partridge Family
28. The Monkees
29. Family Affair
30. All in the Family

31. The Jeffersons
32. One Day at a Time
33. Three's Company
34. Too Close for Comfort
35. Good Times
36. Taxi
37. WKRP
38. The Bob Newhart Show
39. The Love Boat
40. Fantasy Island
41. The Dukes of Hazzard
42. Peter Gunn
43. 77 Sunset Strip
44. Surfside Six
45. Mannix
46. Dragnet
47. Police Story
48. Miami Vice
49. The Blue Knight
50. Hawaii 5-0
51. Police Woman
52. Heart to Heart
53. Black Sheep Squadron
54. MASH
55. Star Trek
56. Marcus Welby
57. Quincy
58. Lassie
59. My Friend Flicka
60. Sky King
61. Perry Mason
62. Ironsides
63. The Waltons
64. Eight Is Enough
65. Little House on the Prairie
66. Bonanza
67. Gunsmoke
68. The Rifleman
69. Wyatt Earp
70. The Virginian
71. The Big Valley
72. As the World Turns
73. General Hospital
74. The Edge of Night
75. The Doctors
76. The Secret Storm
77. Peyton Place
78. Dallas
79. Sixty Minutes
80. The Wild Kingdom
81. American Bandstand
82. The Mickey Mouse Club
83. The Walt Disney Show
84. The Ed Sullivan Show
85. The Carol Burnett Show
86. The Jackie Gleason Show
87. The Phil Silvers Show
88. Donnie and Marie
89. Sonny and Cher
90. Rowan & Martin's Laugh-In
91. Hee Haw
92. Saturday Night Live
93. Johnny Carson
94. David Letterman
95. Phil Donahue
96. Mike Douglas
97. Candid Camera
98. You Bet Your Life (Groucho Marx)
99. Queen for a Day
100. Password
101. The Match Game
102. To Tell the Truth
103. Let's Make a Deal
104. Jeopardy
105. Hollywood Squares
106. Name That Tune
107. Wheel of Fortune

(Note: The game above may be started at one meeting and continued at the next, depending on time considerations.)

Game Six

Try to list as many different breeds of dog as possible.

1. Afghan hound
2. Alaskan husky (Cue: Sled dog)
3. Basset hound
4. Beagle
5. Black lab
6. Brittany spaniel
7. Bulldog
8. Chihuahua (Cue: Mexican)
9. Cockapoo
10. Cocker spaniel
11. Collie (Cue: Lassie)
12. Dachshund (Cue: Sometimes called a "hotdog")
13. Dalmation (Cue: Rides on the fire engine)
14. Doberman (Cue: Known as a good watchdog)
15. Elk hound
16. English setter
17. German shepherd (Cue: Also known as the police dog)
18. Golden lab
19. Golden retriever
20. Great Dane
21. Greyhound (Cue: Known for speed)
22. Irish setter (Cue: Red fur)
23. Malamute
24. Pekingese
25. Pit bull
26. Pointer
27. Poodle
28. Rottweiler
29. St. Bernard (Cue: Known for rescues in the snow)
30. Schnauzer
31. Scottish terrier
32. Spitz
33. Weimaraner
34. Wolf hound

Game Seven

Try to list as many past and present countries of the world as possible.

1. Afghanistan
2. Algeria
3. Argentina

4. Austria
5. Bangladesh
6. Belgium
7. Bermuda (Cue: In the summer you might wear *what* shorts?)
8. Brazil (Cue: A large tasty nut)
9. Cambodia
10. Canada (Cue: Mounties, lumberjacks)
11. Chile
12. China (Cue: Checkers)
13. Colombia
14. Costa Rica
15. Cuba (Cue: Havana cigars)
16. Denmark
17. Dominican Republic
18. Ecuador
19. Egypt (Cue: Pyramids)
20. England
21. Ethiopia
22. Finland
23. France
24. Germany
25. Greece (Cue: Mythological gods)
26. Greenland
27. Guatemala
28. Holland (Cue: Wooden shoes)
29. Haiti
30. Hungary
31. Iceland
32. India (Cue: Sacred cows)
33. Iran
34. Iraq
35. Ireland (Cue: Leprechauns)
36. Israel (Cue: The Jewish nation)
37. Italy (Cue: Spaghetti)
38. Japan
39. Jordan
40. Kenya
41. Korea
42. Laos
43. Lebanon
44. Liberia
45. Libya

46. Lithuania
47. Luxemburg
48. Mexico (Cue: Hat dance; siestas)
49. Monaco (Cue: Princess Grace Kelly)
50. Morocco
51. Netherlands
52. New Zealand
53. Nicaragua
54. Norway
55. Pakistan
56. Panama (Cue: Home of a famous canal)
57. Paraguay
58. Peru
59. Poland
60. Portugal
61. Rumania
62. Russia
63. Saudi Arabia
64. Siam (Cue: Joined twins)
65. Spain (Cue: Bull fights)
66. Sweden (Cue: Known for saunas and massage)
67. Switzerland (Cue: A neutral nation; known for making clocks)
68. Syria
69. Thailand
70. Tibet
71. Turkey
72. Uruguay
73. Venezuela
74. Vietnam

Game Eight

Try to list everything that you would be likely to find on a downtown square or main street. (Cue: Have students think about the services and purchases they might go into town for.)

1. Drug store
2. Dime store
3. Dollar store
4. Card shop
5. Hardware store
6. Florist shop
7. Print shop
8. Jewelry store
9. Pawn shop
10. Furniture store
11. Book store
12. Grocery store
13. Thrift shop
14. Gym
15. Restaurant
16. Coffee shop
17. Pub
18. Barber shop
19. Hairdresser
20. Bank
21. Savings & Loan
22. Finance company
23. Surveyor's office
24. Lawyer's office
25. Newspaper office
26. Radio station
27. Telephone company office
28. Electric company office
29. Gas company office
30. Public library
31. Recreation center
32. Post Office
33. Chamber of Commerce
34. Courthouse
35. Police station
36. Fire station
37. Sidewalks
38. Newspaper stands
39. Bus stops
40. Park benches
41. Parking lots
42. Parking meters
43. Traffic signs
44. Traffic lights

Game Nine

Think of as many professions as possible.

1. Acrobat
2. Actor/actress
3. Animal trainer
4. Architect/draftsman
5. Artist/sculptor
6. Apartment manager
7. Astronaut
8. Babysitter/nanny
9. Banker/teller
10. Barber/beautician
11. Bartender
12. Boat captain
13. Bookkeeper/accountant
14. Builder/carpenter/contractor
15. Busdriver
16. Butler
17. Cabdriver
18. Cashier
19. Clown
20. Coin collector/art collector
21. Cook/chef
22. Dancer
23. Delivery man
24. Dentist
25. Detective
26. Dietitian

27. Doctor
28. Editor
29. Electrician
30. Engineer
31. Exercise instructor
32. Farmer
33. File clerk
34. Fireman
35. Fisherman
36. Florist
37. Garbage collector
38. Gardener
39. Gym coach/football coach
40. Hobo
41. Horticulturist
42. Housekeeper/maid
43. House painter
44. Hypnotist
45. Indian chief
46. Insurance agent
47. Interior decorator
48. Journalist
49. Land surveyor
50. Lawyer
51. Librarian
52. Lifeguard
53. Magician
54. Mailman
55. Maintenance man
56. Matador
57. Mechanic
58. Model
59. Mortician
60. Nurse
61. Optician/ophthalmologist
62. Pharmacist
63. Photographer
64. Pilot
65. Plumber

66. Policeman
67. Politician
68. Priest/minister/nun/monk/rabbi
69. Printer
70. Professor
71. Proofreader
72. Psychologist
73. Radio announcer/TV announcer
74. Real estate agent
75. Retail store manager
76. Salesman/traveling salesman
77. Schoolteacher
78. Scientist
79. Seamstress
80. Secretary/receptionist
81. Singer
82. Soldier
83. Sports professional/athlete
84. Spy
85. Stockbroker
86. Telephone operator
87. Tightrope walker
88. Travel agent
89. Truckdriver
90. Typist
91. Veterinarian
92. Waiter/waitress
93. Wild game hunter
94. Writer

(Note: The game above may be started at one meeting and continued at the next, depending on time considerations.)

Game Ten

Try to list as many words and items possible that are associated with falling in love. (Cue: Ask questions such as: "What would a bride wear?" "What might the bride toss to her attendants?" and, "What might the couple drink to make a toast?")

1. Dating
2. Holding hands
3. Hugging
4. Kissing
5. Girlfriend
6. Boyfriend
7. Hearts
8. Sweethearts
9. Valentines
10. Cards
11. Poems
12. Candy
13. Flowers
14. Sweet talk
15. Promises
16. Getting "pinned"
17. Getting engaged/proposal
18. Engagement ring
19. Wedding band
20. Bridal showers
21. Bridal parties
22. Rehearsal party
23. Proxy or stand-in
24. Bride and groom
25. Church/courthouse
26. Minister/judge
27. Wedding gown
28. Veil
29. Tuxedo
30. Bridesmaids
31. Maid or matron of honor
32. Ushers
33. Best man
34. Flower girl
35. Ring bearer
36. Mother of the bride
37. Mother of the groom
38. Corsages
39. Floral decorations
40. Throwing the bouquet
41. Something old, new, borrowed, and blue
42. Ornate garter
43. Giving away the bride
44. Crying at the wedding
45. Kissing the bride
46. Decorating the car
47. Wedding cake
48. Refreshments
49. Champagne
50. Dancing
51. Wedding gifts
52. Honeymoon
53. Husband and wife
54. Starting a family
55. Anniversaries

Summary

The games described in this chapter will suggest other similar types of mental fitness games that you can play with your students. You might, for example, conduct the Amen Game using hit Broadway shows, presidents of the United States, or other historical characters and facts.

Don't try to structure List Game activities too rigidly. If I have listed forty possible answers for a given game, your group may come up with twenty or they may come up with fifty. Naturally, they shouldn't be restricted to listing items in any specific order.

Below are some examples of additional List Game topics that have proven fun and stimulating for my nursing home fitness students:

1) List makes and models of automobiles
2) List items that you would be likely to find in a kitchen
3) List famous actors, actresses, and singers
4) List names for girls
5) List different kinds of flowers
6) List all your favorite foods
7) List all the things that a person might wear
8) List things that are associated with Christmas
9) List specific brand names (such as Betty Crocker, Maybelline, Ivory, Del Monte, Bounty, Jergens, etc.)
10) List places that make good vacation spots, the activities that you might expect to enjoy there, and the sights that you would expect to see.

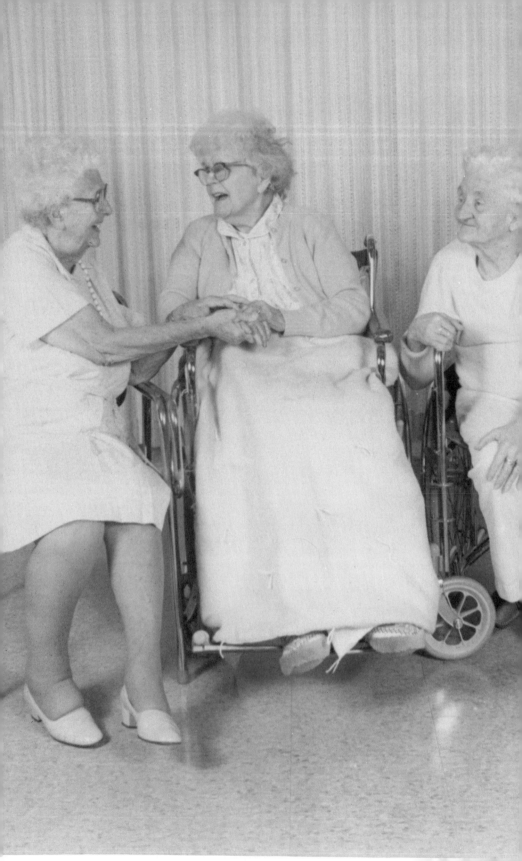

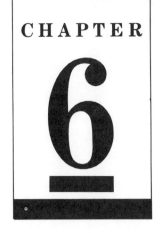

CHAPTER 6

Group Discussions for Mental Fitness

Whether you have a group of twenty or just one student and a leader, discussion activity adds the benefits of social interaction to intellectual exercise. Discussion should be conducted during the segment of the Seniorcise class that has been set aside for a mental fitness activity.

Key Principles

The following guidelines will help you, first, to get your group discussion started and, second, to keep the sharing and conversation flowing.

1) Try to select topics that will give rise to pleasant, discussable memories for your students — not to sad or highly personal memories.

2) When phrasing a discussion topic proposal, do not use superlatives such as: "Tell us about the *happiest* moment of your *life*," or "Tell us the *funniest* joke you *ever* heard." That will place unnecessary pressure on the student and make it harder for him to think. Instead, try: "Think back to a happy occasion in your past," or, "Let's try to remember some jokes." By keeping the scope of your discussion broader and more general, you will help to ensure the student's success. Since you have not limited him to one unsurpassed experience, he may even be able to relate several memories on the same subject.

3) Come prepared to make several contributions on the topic yourself. You will probably need to present one or two ideas at the beginning of the discussion in order to start the ball rolling. You might, for example, say: "I remember an especially happy day ten years ago. It was my wedding day!" This should remind members of their own family weddings, births, baptisms, and bar mitzvahs.

Later on during the same discussion, you might need to introduce a new direction to prompt further thought among the students. At that point you could say: "I remember another happy time a few years back. My husband won us two hundred dollars in a sweepstakes! Have any of you ever won a drawing or a contest?"

4) If your examples fail to stir the memories you'd hoped for among your students, then make suggestions directly: "Babies often bring joy and happiness. Who can remember a very welcomed arrival in their family?"

5) Since new blood can help to stimulate conversation, be sure to include guests and volunteer assistants in your group discussions. If a staff member passes by at an opportune moment, ask if he has time to contribute something on the subject.

6) Members will feel freer to respond if you keep the atmosphere casual during discussion periods. You can help to put students at ease by using informal phrases such as: "See if you can remember back to a time . . ."; "Tell us a little about . . ."; "Let's have a pow-wow about . . ."; and, "For today's *tete-a-tete* . . ." You can still incorporate a sense of challenge, for example, by saying: "I'll tell a story on myself if you'll tell a story on yourself!"

7) Use facts that you already know about a student to draw him out during discussions. Say, for example: "Bill, I understand that you were reunited with your twin brother after twenty years of separation. That must have been a pretty happy moment for you both! Could you describe it for us?" (Note: Your discussion about happy moments may now lead to a discussion about twins. Don't interfere with the direction a discussion takes as long as your members are following and enjoying it. If they reach a stalemate, guide them back to the last point of reference: "Finding his twin was a happy moment for Bill. Who else can remember a happy moment to share with us?")

8) If a student can't remember a personal experience of his own, encourage him to talk about a relative or an acquaintance. Likewise, a certain topic may leave *you* at a loss for words. In that case, you might say: "My neighbors had a happy experience. Their five-year-old son had wandered deep into the woods behind their house. He was missing overnight, and they were frantic with worry. The next morning a state trooper found him curled up asleep beside a log. Boy, were his parents happy when he came home safe and sound." Or, use the examples I've included in this chapter: "I heard about a lady who . . ."

9) Once a student does begin talking, hush up and LISTEN. Don't interrupt. And don't fill in words for him if he pauses to collect his thoughts mid-story. Encourage all of your members to give each speaker in turn their undivided attention. If a student's voice is not strong enough to be heard by the others, repeat his story to them after he has finished.

10) Bring your group discussion to a tidy close by restating the topic, providing a brief recap of the material discussed, and thanking the students

who made contributions. You might say: "It was fun talking over some of the happy experiences we've had. We learned about Bill's reunion with his brother and about Ed's return home after the war. We heard about Mary's wedding and about the birth of Anna's first grandchild. Then there was Helen's debutante ball, and don't let me forget Jack's successes at the race track! Thank you all for sharing your reminiscences."

Group Discussion Topics

Below are ten topic ideas that proved to be favorites at our fitness meetings. Included with each topic are several examples of the kinds of cues you can employ to get specific discussions started and to keep them going.

Discussion One

Try to remember a time when someone did something especially nice for you.

Cue Examples:

1) "No one can remember one right off the bat? That's OK. Maybe this will remind you of one. Last year my car broke down completely. I bought another one, but it was a lemon. It was in the shop so much that I had to walk to work every day. I was tired all the time. But then my dad loaned me his car. He said to keep it for as long as I needed it. I'll tell you, it really helped me out. Did anyone ever come to your rescue like that?"

2) "Did everyone hear Alice's story? After attending a big family reunion, she fell as she was getting into her car. But her nephew ran right over, helped her up, and saw that she got home safely. She really appreciated that."

3) "I just remembered another nice thing someone did for me. When I got married, my fiance and I paid for our own wedding. We didn't have much money to start our new lives together with, so we decided to be extra thrifty. We weren't going to have a reception party after the ceremony. But a dear friend provided a lovely party for everyone with flowers, cake, sandwiches, and champagne! That really meant a lot to us. Has anyone ever given a party for you? Maybe on your birthday?"

4) "Louise just made a good point. She said that the nurses help her with her bath every day. Can anyone think of other nice things that the nurses and aids here do?"

5) "Let's add a new twist to this discussion. Try to remember when you did something especially nice for another person. Betty, I know you have twenty-two grandchildren and that you have helped your children many times by babysitting. What's it like to have such a large family calling on your services?"

Discussion Two

Try to remember a time when your pet (or an animal that you owned) got you into trouble.

Cue Examples:

1) "Boy, you all must have had well-behaved pets! Let me tell you what my cat Hal did. He's a very big cat, and he's always under my feet. One day I was running to answer the telephone, and I tripped over him. I went sailing through the air, crashed into the dining room table, and broke my nose. I had to go straight to the hospital emergency room. Needless to say, I never did make it to the phone or find out who was trying to call me. Now who can top that story?"

2) "That same cat Hal bit my sister-in-law. I was so embarrassed. Would you believe I still have this cat? Did any of you ever have an animal that bit somebody?"

3) "Bob, I know that you once ran a big dairy farm, and I'll bet those cattle broke down the fence every now and then. What did you do when a bunch of cows got out into the road?"

4) "That was a great story, Margaret. I bet your mother got mad when your puppy stole her pie off the window sill. Animals do love food, don't they? Did anyone else's pet ever steal a snack?"

5) "I had a dog named Blackie who took a liking to welcome mats. Every night he stole another neighbor's welcome mat and brought it home. At one point I had twenty welcome mats at my front door! What would you do if your dog brought home twenty stolen welcome mats?"

6) "I heard a story about a dog named Lightnin'. Lightnin' used to jump over the fence in her yard and then go up and down the street destroying every piece of plastic lawn furniture she could find. The neighbors complained so much that her owner had to build a higher fence. Have any of you ever known a dog that loved to chew up things?"

Discussion Three

Try to remember a time when you laughed so hard you thought you would cry.

Cue Examples:

1) "Sometimes something is funny simply because it is so unexpected. For instance, a friend and I thought we were going to hear an amusing talk by a famous cartoonist. After we sat down, it slowly dawned on us that we had gotten ourselves into a very boring lecture on South American agricultural methods. Everyone else in the room was listening and taking notes in dead earnest. But every time my friend and I met eyes, we couldn't help but burst

into laughter. Then all those serious people would turn around and look at us in irritation, and that would only make it even harder for us to stop laughing! Have you ever gotten yourself into a similar predicament?"

2) "Carl's story about hiding the rubber snake in his teacher's lunchbox should remind us of other pranks we thought were funny during our school days."

3) "In a way, Edna's story about laughing out loud in school is like my story about laughing during that serious lecture. Have you ever noticed that things seem funnier in places where you're not supposed to laugh? Let's take church, for instance. We all know that we should be quiet and reverent at church. But did anything ever happen to crack you up during a church service?"

4) "Paul, I know that you spent a few years working in a traveling carnival. With all those interesting characters about — the bearded lady, the fortune teller, the thin man, and the clowns — there must have been some pretty funny incidents. Tell us a little bit about those days."

5) "Peggy, that's a terrific example. Red Skelton actually made her laugh till she cried when she saw his live show. Has anyone else seen a funny comedian either in person or on TV?"

6) "How about jokes and riddles? Have you heard any that really struck your funny bone? Let's try to remember some now. Did you hear the one about . . ."

Discussion Four
Think back to a time when you felt especially close to nature.

Cue Examples:
1) "I grew up on a farm. When I was a girl, I used to love to go out into the middle of a pasture and lie on my back in the tall grass. No one knew where I was, and it was very quiet. All I could see was the green grass around me and the blue sky above. I'll never forget how peaceful it was. Have you ever enjoyed just being alone in your own secret outdoor refuge?"

2) "Laura is right. Discovering that waterfall during her walk must have made her feel very close to nature. Who else has gone hiking before?"

3) "Jerry, I think that a lot of people will agree with you. He says that being in the mountains makes him feel closer to nature than being anywhere else does. What gives the rest of you a closer feeling to nature, the mountains or the beach?"

4) "Another time that I felt particularly close to nature was while swimming at a beach in Georgia. I had been so busy trying to make a living in Atlanta that I had not been to see the ocean for four years. As soon as I saw it again, I had to jump in! Have any of you ever gotten so wrapped

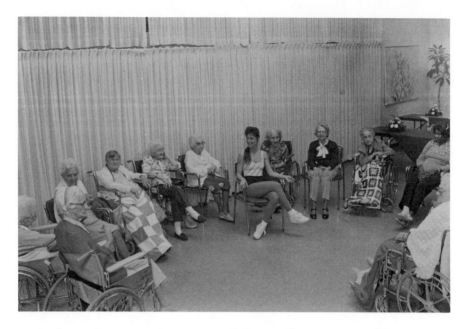

up in day-to-day cares that you needed to rediscover nature?"

5) "Speaking of Atlanta, there were some lovely parks there right in the middle of the city. Jim, I know you come from Chicago. Tell us about its parks and natural attractions."

6) "Now, I know that some of you grew up way out in the country just like I did. And I can't believe you didn't know every swimming hole within ten miles of your front doors! Didn't you ever tie a rope to a tree limb so you could swing out and jump in the water? You country folks, put on your thinking caps!"

7) "Alma felt close to nature when she fed the raccoons that lived in her yard. Has anyone here ever kept a birdfeeder?"

Discussion Five

Try to remember a time when you worked so hard you thought you might drop.

Cue Examples:

1) "That's an easy one for me. When I was growing up in South Carolina I used to pick cotton in a neighbor's fields. We carried the cotton in croker sacks and got paid by the bushel. Boy, did it ever get hot sometimes! Anyone else ever pick cotton? Anyone ever grow a garden?"

2) "Ben, you were in the Navy, weren't you? What types of jobs did you have to do as a sailor?"

3) "You know, moving is hard work. Did anyone ever move from one part

of the country to another?"

4) "Rearing children can be hard work. Betty, you should know since you had eight! How did you manage all those kids?"

5) "Ted, I know you were in the newspaper business. Now it seems like that would be pretty tough work with all those deadlines to meet every day. What was it really like?"

Discussion Six
Try to remember an embarrassing moment in your past.

Cue Examples:

1) "I know it's a hard topic, but maybe this will remind you of an embarrassing moment. When I was twelve I appeared in a piano recital. I knew my piece by heart, of course. But when I got up in front of all those people, I got so nervous that I completely forgot it. Has anyone else ever lost his wits when he had to speak or perform before a group?"

2) "Now come on! I told you an embarrassing story about myself, so now you should tell one, too. Be fair!"

3) "Thank you for contributing to our discussion, Nurse Johnson. We won't tell anyone about the hook on your swimsuit breaking! Have any of you ever seen that happen to someone?"

4) "I once heard a story about a famous art museum that was giving a show of modern art. One of the artists complained that his work had been hung upside down. The curator's face was really red!"

5) "Pat says that she has seen cats get embarrassed. After missing a jump, they seem to pretend that they fell on purpose. Now isn't that just like us people?"

6) "I guess John just gave the classic example of the ultimate embarrassing moment. Has anyone else's mind ever gone completely blank while introducing someone — a person whose name you've known for years?"

7) "Our social lives can get complicated, and that sometimes leads to embarrassing situations. Did anyone ever accidentally line up two dates for the same evening? Any of you ladies ever go to a party where another woman had on a dress exactly like yours?"

Discussion Seven
Try to remember a show that you enjoyed watching.

Cue Examples:

1) "Sometimes we enjoy shows that we don't expect to enjoy. I'm a rock 'n' roll fan myself, so when I went to see Carol Channing's live show with my parents I thought I'd be bored. But that lady has so much stage presence

she actually had me sitting on the edge of my seat!"

2) "Remember when Peggy told us about seeing Red Skelton perform in person? I've seen Carol Channing, Elvis, and several others. Who else has been to a live performance or concert?"

3) "Who can remember attending a play?"

4) "Linda, you're from New York City. Did you ever visit Broadway?"

5) "What about movies? I love *Gone With the Wind*. And I bet there are some Humphrey Bogart fans in here. Who remembers watching a good movie?"

6) "Rachel, you played the piano in your husband's dance band for years. So you *were* the show, weren't you? Tell us what it was like being on stage."

7) "Well, I happen to remember a good show that every one of you saw. Remember when the breakdancers came here and danced for us? What did you think about the music they used?"

Discussion Eight

Think back to a moment when you felt very proud of yourself.

Cue Examples:

1) "I was proud — and relieved — when I passed the entrance exam to get into graduate school. Does anyone else remember passing a difficult test?"

2) "Henry, I understand that you played pro baseball for a while. I bet you were proud when you made the team."

3) "Winning an election might make someone feel proud. Has anyone here ever been elected president of a club or organization?"

4) "Ed, didn't you receive a military medal? What type of an award was that?"

5) "Marvin said he was proud when he earned promotions at work. And Lois was proud of her husband when he earned promotions. I bet some of you have been proud of your children, too. Does anyone remember attending a son or daughter's high school graduation?"

6) "Who won our wheelchair race last week?"

7) "Many United States citizens are proud to be Americans. Does anyone here get a lump in his throat when 'The Star-Spangled Banner' is played? How do you feel when you see the stars and stripes?"

Discussion Nine

Try to remember a time when you ate too much.

Cue Examples:

1) "When I was in the third grade, my best friend and I ate a whole box

of homemade mints. We both got sick, and to this day I still can't look at a mint! Has anyone else ever gotten carried away eating candy?"

2) "Cindy, you mentioned working at an ice cream parlor. Did you ever get tired of ice cream?"

3) "Think back to some of those big, family Thanksgiving dinners."

4) "What about covered-dish suppers?"

5) "Has anyone ever been to a pie-eating contest?"

6) "What about all-you-can-eat specials at your favorite restaurant?"

7) "Sometimes our eyes are bigger than our stomachs. One time at a cafeteria, everything looked so good that I piled my plate high. I ate so much I could hardly move, but I still couldn't finish it all. Has that ever happened to you in a cafeteria?"

8) "I heard that there were plenty of hotdogs at the picnic you all went on recently. Tell me about that trip. Where did you go? What was the weather like? (etc.)"

Discussion Ten

Try to remember a place you visited that made a special impression on you.

Cue Examples:

1) "I toured the Biltmore House in Asheville, North Carolina. It is a huge mansion that looks like a castle. Has anyone ever seen a palace?"

2) "Sometimes a place is intriguing because of its history — Washington, D.C., for example."

3) "A place can be interesting because of the people who settled it — Chinatown, for example."

4) "Architecture can help to make a city special. I love the old streets and houses in Savannah, Georgia."

5) "Sometimes a place is particularly memorable due to the type of work carried on there. Tarpon Springs, Florida, for instance, is an old Greek sponging village."

6) "One place that I truly fell in love with was Quebec City in Canada. Who else has visited a foreign country?"

7) "Roger, I'm sorry to say that I've never visited your hometown, San Francisco. But I hear that it is a beautiful, hilly city. Could you tell us a little bit about it?"

Conclusion

The more you talk with your students, the better you will get to know them. And the better you get to know your students, the easier it becomes to conduct group discussions. Before long, you will be able to plan discussion topics based on your knowledge of your students' interests and experiences.

Below are five additional topics designed to help you get to know students better and to conduct enthusiastic group discussions simultaneously:

1) A time you got lost;

2) A fear you overcame;

3) A bad habit you overcame (or a difficult challenge that you met);

4) A time when you got all dressed up and looked terrific;

5) A saying or rule that your parents drilled into you when you were growing up.

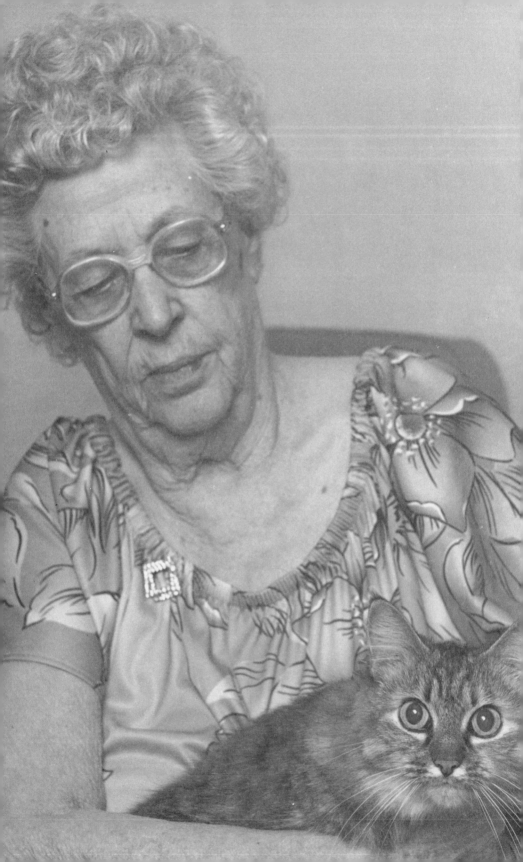

CHAPTER

7

Working with the Elderly One-on-One

If you are caring for an elderly relative at home you may have experienced doubts about how to help him occupy himself in a rewarding manner. If you frequently call on a loved one who lives in a nursing facility you may have wondered if there were more productive ways to pass the time during your visits. If you are a group fitness leader at a nursing facility you may have met certain residents who would benefit from your program but who are unable to attend class for physical or psychological reasons. All of these cases call for the application of a custom-designed fitness program for the solitary elderly individual.

On one level, when you establish a routine of meeting and working together with a single student you will help to alleviate any chronic feelings of loneliness or alienation he may harbor. Every time he accepts a challenge from you he will place a demand upon himself and that, in turn, will serve to make his life fuller and more meaningful.

On another level, when you play simple intellectual games with a person who spends a great deal of time alone you will provide him with additional means and incentive to keep his mental abilities keen. Furthermore, the personal nature of a one-on-one relationship gives you many opportunities to encourage that person to pursue mental stimulation on his own, for example, by working crossword puzzles.

On a strictly physical level, exercising with the single student helps him to realize the same gains that group students realize, such as preventing muscle atrophy and losses in range of motion. Exercising is a practical way to nurture your student's independence, for example through maintaining his ability to bend over and pick up something that has fallen to the floor.

At Home

If your schedule is flexible, meet with your student during the time of day that he is at his brightest. If finding *any* time is a problem for you, then enlist the help of family members in conducting your program. Set up a system of taking turns. In many families there will be children capable of taking part, also. If so, the elderly relative is sure to enjoy their participation. Do try to space out at least three meetings during every week.

Ask your student's physician to look over the exercise directions provided in Chapter Two of this book. He is in a position to know if any particular movement is not recommended for your student. But it is more likely that he will be able to suggest additional exercises especially beneficial in view of your student's overall health.

In conducting a fitness program at home you will have many advantages that a nursing home fitness leader lacks. You will have more days per week from which to select meeting times. You can concentrate all of your attention on one student. Your bonds of kinship and the years of shared love will help to motivate and support you in your efforts. Meanwhile, your intimate knowledge of the student will aid you in planning activities that he will enjoy, in selecting game and discussion topics that will interest him, and in providing cues that will relate to his experiences.

There are several predictable obstacles that you might encounter in trying to set up an at-home fitness program. Perhaps you will feel ill-prepared or unsure of yourself in the role of fitness leader. If you do have misgivings or questions, don't be too shy to ask for a little help. You might, for example, call your local nursing home and ask to speak to the activities coordinator or to the fitness instructor. Either one should be able to address your specific questions and might also offer some additional advice to help you get off to a good start.

Better yet, you may be able to arrange a visit to the nursing home in order to observe a group fitness meeting in progress (just don't be surprised if you get "put to work" playing ball or keeping a scoreboard during your visit!). If the nursing home has a one-on-one program, you may be permitted to accompany the fitness instructor on his rounds. This experience would most closely simulate your projected at-home program. While you are at the nursing home, you will see the equipment used during fitness activities. The fitness instructor can tell you where it is sold and how much it costs. He may also suggest other resources such as books, cassette tapes, or video tapes appropriate to your circumstances. When you visit the nursing home, be sure to carry a notepad so you can jot down facts and ideas that may be useful later. Once you've been to the nursing home to see a little, do a little, and talk a little with an experienced geriatric fitness leader, you are bound to feel more confident about trying it on your own.

Another hurdle you may have to overcome to establish an at-home fitness program is the resistance of an elderly person who does not see any need to exercise. Perhaps you come from a family in which the value of physical exercise was never stressed. Or, perhaps your elderly loved one was physically active all of his life up until the stroke (or, up until the broken hip, the amputation, the operation . . .) but now he is saying that he is old, he deserves a rest, and he can see no reason why he shouldn't rest for the remainder of his days. This can be a very difficult problem. It must be stated from the outset without any ifs, buts, or ands that a person — no matter how good his intentions — cannot make another person exercise. Fitness is elective. Like anyone else, an elderly person has every right to refuse it. His rights must be respected. And that is that.

If, however, your exercise candidate is willing to discuss the idea, even though he honestly just doesn't see what is to be gained, then you are in a tenable position. You should be prepared to state practical, good-sense reasons for following a program of regular exercise. Draw upon the preceding chapters of this book, which contain many examples of daily tasks that exercise can facilitate. Grip performance has been discussed (important for maintaining the ability to hold drinking glasses, writing utensils, and other hand-held objects). Coordination has been discussed (important for *manipulating* hand-held objects and for negotiating one's way through doors and around corners). Strength has been cited (important for getting up out of bed or up from a chair, or for lifting a book). Flexibility, or range of motion, has also been considered. (Remember? We need it for getting that sweater on and also when bending or reaching for objects.) Many of the exercises described in Chapter Two are designed to improve one's skeletal muscle endurance. This type of muscular ability is useful for sustaining pleasant activities such as knitting and for accomplishing repetitive movements such as self-pushing a wheelchair or advancing a portable walker.

If your Doubting Thomas remains unconvinced that an exercise program will do him good, then ask his doctor to talk with him. As previously stated, medical approval must be obtained before starting the program anyway. So, perhaps you can kill two birds with one stone. The doctor will know that prolonged disuse results in muscle atrophy, reductions in range of motion, and declines in muscular strength and endurance. He can effectively counter any misconceptions, such as: "I can't do it" or "It's too late to start exercising now." His encouragement could make all the difference. Indeed, he may add a schedule of walking (or assisted walking) to the program if he feels it is indicated.

When working with an elderly relative, especially one of your parents, you may feel awkward about making suggestions or trying to help direct his activities. If so, then try making fitness a joint project. Ask him to do the workouts *with* you as opposed to *for* you. If you already exercise regularly, the addition of light, seated calisthenics will complement your regimen without constituting a strain. However, chances are that you have not been finding the time for adequate exercise recently. Performing these gentle Seniorcise workouts will be a good way to ease yourself back into an exercise lifestyle. By using this approach, the two of you can help each other. Always proceed at your elderly relative's pace, and keep a written record (together, if possible) of his progress, being sure to log in important advances. For example, note when repetitions are increased, when new exercises are learned, or when light resistance is added. A written reminder of past achievements may help to inspire perseverance later if his motivation begins to flag.

The same approach can be used when trying to interest your elderly loved one in mental fitness activities. First of all, get interested yourself! Nowadays, it is just too easy to flop in front of the television instead of providing our intellects with more demanding pursuits. At any rate, one thing is for certain — tackling a simple puzzle won't do any of us a bit of harm. So, why not undertake mental fitness activities together? You might, for example, suggest, "Let's get some mental stimulation today. I'd like to work on this list game. Will you help me?" From your point of view, it may

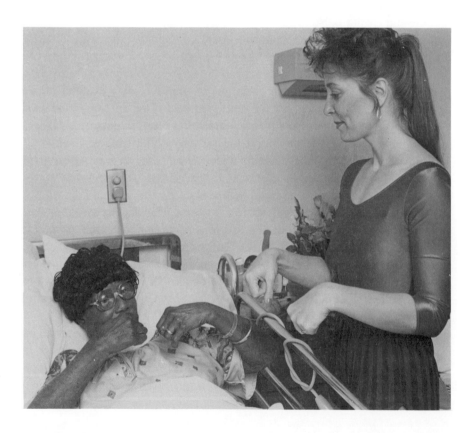

well prove to be more stimulating — and more fun — than you expected.

Fun, in fact, should be given high priority in your at-home geriatric fitness program. If your elderly loved one can look forward to meetings which he knows are going to be pleasurable, the stage will be set for willing participation and success. So, take the necessary steps to keep your meetings relaxed and enjoyable. Try to prevent minor household interruptions. Set aside other times for discussing business or family matters. Make each meeting a special time for you and your elderly relative — a time to enjoy just being together, a time to focus on fitness and fun.

In a Facility

The number of single students that you can serve as a nursing home fitness leader will, of necessity, depend on the amount of time you have available and on the facility's financial budget if you are a paid employee. The nursing home activities coordinator should be able to recommend residents for one-on-one work and to secure written medical approval of their participation.

As a rule, the student assigned to you as an individual subject will be one who does not attend other nursing home activities. Consequently, you will

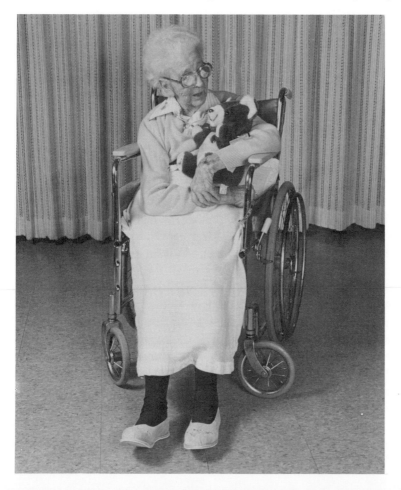

probably know very little, if anything, about him. A good way to begin his program is to talk with the nurse in charge of his hall. She can give you a rundown of the information on his medical chart. She can also advise you on his present ability to exercise, his physical potential, his emotional state, and the degree of cooperation you can expect to receive from his family.

The involvement of family members who visit your private student can be very helpful. Concerned relatives have bought Nerf balls for my single students to exercise with and stuffed toys for them to carry, squeeze, and hug (which uses muscles, also). They have learned to supervise the exercises on days when I wasn't scheduled to visit their loved ones.

Remember that aids and maintenance personnel see your student almost every day. They might be able to share insights that will prove valuable in planning his fitness program. Keep aware, however, of their hectic work schedules. They may have been directed to assist you — for instance, if you request that a student be lifted from his bed to his wheelchair for a meeting. And they will *want* to assist you, too. But don't make their work more difficult by constantly arriving just when they're trying to change bed pans, serve meals, or mop floors.

In General

Whether your one-on-one fitness program is conducted at home or in an institutional setting, it must incorporate two essential ingredients in order to be successful. These essential elements are communication and creativity. The following examples demonstrate their value.

Ray

Ray was extremely intelligent and well-spoken. He had injured his spine in a boating accident and was left with little use of his arms and legs. His doctors had recently terminated physical therapy, stating that it was useless. Under the circumstances, Ray was not eager to embark on a fitness program of any description. But instead of removing his name from my case load, the activities coordinator suggested that I continue to drop in on Ray — not to exercise, but just to talk. During one visit he expressed concern over the abdominal fat he had gained thanks to all the enforced inactivity. So I spoke to his former physical therapist, who assured me that trying to perform situps in bed would not hurt Ray.

"But will they help?" I wondered. The therapist told me to place my palm on Ray's abdomen and ask him to cough. If the rectus abdominis contracted (that is, the *outer* muscle, not the deeply located diaphragm), then I should assume that it had the potential to benefit from exercise.

The muscle did contract, and Ray began a program of situps. Before long he was performing biceps curls too, and later we added other exercises.

Marcia

Marcia was the youngest resident of the nursing home. At forty, she had recently suffered a stroke that left her paralyzed on the left side of her body. The doctor's prognosis was favorable. Although she could not expect to regain the use of her left limbs, she could look forward to otherwise good health and she could regain her speech abilities through voice therapy.

The nurses encouraged Marcia to attend group fitness class, but she refused because she was so much younger than the other students. They encouraged her to work towards her speech goals, too. But Marcia continued to feel more frustrated than motivated.

When Marcia was assigned to me for one-on-one fitness classes I noticed that, like so many students, she responded best to ball activities. So the administrator of the nursing home approved the purchase of a Nerf ball for Marcia's private use. She was pleased with the ball, but never used it without supervision because it invariably got away from her and she could not retrieve it. Finally it occurred to me to customize the ball to her needs. Using a large needle, I worked a string through the ball and knotted one end so that it would stay. Now she could tie the ball to her wheelchair whenever she liked and pull it back by its string when she lost it.

Being able to exercise control over the ball worked wonders in Marcia's attitude. Soon she was applying herself with greater energy towards regaining both her strength and her speech.

Luke

Another stroke victim, Luke suffered from severe emotional problems as well. Too frightened and shy to attend group class, Luke was as much a recluse as it is possible to be in a busy nursing home. The first few times I visited him, he never even raised his head, which rested on his arm upon a table by his wheelchair. I tried many tactics to get Luke's attention — humor, for instance: "Come on, Luke. I know you've heard of the Bionic Man. Since you rely on that one good arm, let's make it a bionic arm with exercise!"

Everything failed until an aid told me that before Luke moved to the nursing home he had at one time been an avid gardener. So I brought Luke a pathetic potted plant that had failed to thrive at my house. His interest kindled, Luke nursed the plant back to vitality and began to respond to my exercise suggestions, too.

Setting Goals and Recognizing Progress

The activities coordinator and the medical staff can help you set reasonable goals for your students. In some cases, progress is made when a student takes over some of his own self-grooming tasks, such as brushing his hair.

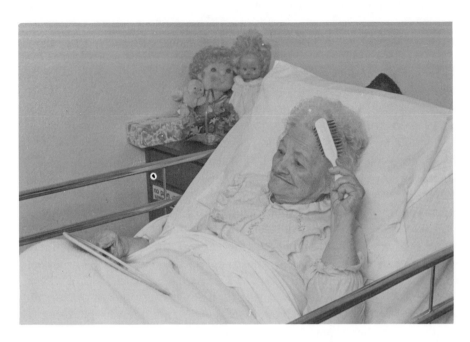

In other cases, it may take weeks before a student begins to remember you from one visit to the next. Do be sure to recognize that advance when it is made.

Set realistic short-term goals. For example, have the student work on learning your name, or help the student to appreciate and to accept regular physical exercise.

The long-term goal that I am requested to work towards most often is this: "Try to get him interested in something. He wants to stay in bed all the time. He needs to get out of his room and be more active." And that is certainly a feasible goal. One student was, in fact, so successful in overcoming her bedridden listlessness that she has since been awarded a wheelchair and now attends our group meetings!

Keep a notebook in which to record short-term and long-term goals. Be sure to chronicle every triumph, no matter how small. It will help you when interested family members or nursing home personnel ask for a progress report on a particular student. A written reminder of former successes will also help you when you need a little psychological boost yourself.

Exercise Activities

All of the exercise activities described in Chapter Two can be adapted from group use to personal use. Pay particular attention to the section of that chapter entitled "Exercising While Standing, Sitting, or Lying Down." And do consider outfitting your private student with his own set of hand-weights to keep in his room. See Chapter Two's section on "Pumping Iron" for specifics.

Ball Activities

Look at the arm and wrist exercises described in the three Seniorcise workouts provided in Chapter Two. Notice that many of these exercises can be performed while holding a Nerf ball in one or both hands.

The waste basket toss and the squeezing exercises described under the section on Nerf Ball Activities provided in Chapter Three work extremely well in a one-on-one program. Bowling and kickball (using an inflatable beachball), also described in Chapter Three, can be enjoyed by two players as well as by a group.

The simple but challenging game of catch (using a Nerf ball) is the overall favorite activity of my one-on-one fitness students. Throw the ball gently so that your student can, if necessary, trap it between his arm and his body. Set goals according to the student's progress, for example: "You've been tossing the ball so well. Let's start working towards catching it, too"; "Last week we kept the game going for five throws and catches. Let's try to break our old record today"; "Let's try for ten in a row"; or, "Let's just count how many times we can keep it going." Your student may enjoy counting aloud with you during play. Be sure to note both goals and accomplishments in your record book.

Sports and Special Activities

Peruse Chapter Four of this book for special events to which you might expose your individual student. If you have a VCR at home, presenting fitness-related videos is a possibility. And a special guest or volunteer assistant is always a pleasant surprise for the solitary student.

Mental Activities

Every intellectual game described in Chapter Five can be played by one student with a leader. As in group class, be sure to explain the purpose of the activity to your private student. Keep the atmosphere relaxed and informal during play. Just sit with your student, and write on a sheet of paper instead of a blackboard. Use a big felt-tipped pen to effect large clear lettering, and hold the paper in a position that your student can easily see.

Likewise, each discussion activity listed in Chapter Six can also be enjoyed by two. Again, don't forget to explain the purpose of the exercise. Then just sit and talk with your student, keeping the mood conversational. Remember

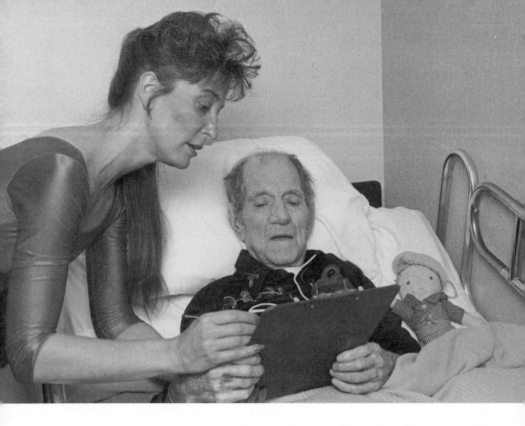

that in working one-on-one with a student, you'll need to be prepared to contribute more than usual to any given discussion, since there will be fewer participants to exchange ideas and memories.

Conclusion

Working individually with an elderly fitness student will give you the opportunity to get to know him very well. You will be able to help him set goals that will effectively improve the quality of his life. As he fulfills these goals, you will experience the satisfaction that comes from helping another to work towards and earn greater personal freedom.

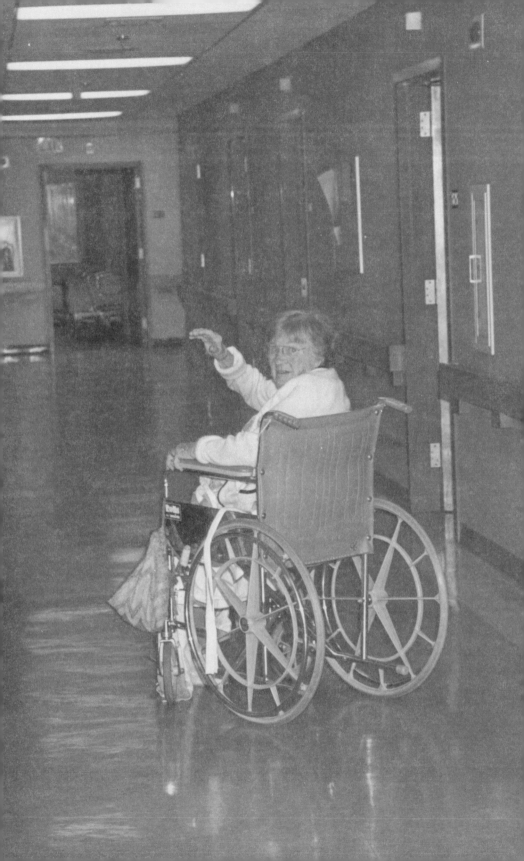

CHAPTER

8

Parting Ways

Various circumstances can result in an active student's departure from your fitness program. But, as his fitness leader, you need not stand by helplessly as he leaves your realm of influence. There are many steps that you can take to help ensure his continued participation and success in a program of mental and physical fitness.

Transfers

One of your students may be transferred to a different nursing home altogether. When this occurs, you can take positive action by telephoning the activities coordinator or the fitness instructor at his new home. In my experience, fellow recreational personnel have always been pleased and extremely cooperative when contacted.

Several objectives can be accomplished by communicating with the student's new fitness leader. First of all, if the leader knows that the student has been active in another fitness program, then the leader will not waver in urging him to join the activities at his new home. By informing the new leader of the student's favorite fitness activities, you will give the leader a tool with which to draw him into the new program. Be sure to volunteer any special knowledge that you have regarding the student which may prove helpful in the application of his fitness program. This advice might include, for example, methods you employed to minimize his physical limitations during class, specific sports or games at which he excelled, or aspects of his personal history that you found relevant for motivational purposes.

Moving to a new environment can be traumatic for anyone, and the elderly fitness student is no exception. In the case of one transfer from our nursing home to another, I was surprised to learn that Ada, an outstanding fitness student, had grown apathetic and was refusing to show an interest in activities offered by her new facility. The reasons were obvious to her new activities coordinator: Ada missed her former friends and longed for her old routine.

In cases like Ada's, establishing contact with an employee of the new facility can expedite the student's adaptation process. The student is likely to start feeling more at home in his new environment when he learns that special steps have been taken to make the transition smoother for him. A connection between his old and new fitness leaders will provide him with a greater sense of continuity and progression. And, the knowledge that his old friends miss him enough to call about his welfare will bolster his self-esteem and make it easier to cultivate new friends.

After her conversation with me, Ada's new activities coordinator was able to deliver cheerful news to her: "The members of your Ocean View fitness class send you a big HELLO. And, the fitness leader there tells me that you're a super kickball player. I just happen to have a new ball that needs breaking in, and I think you're the woman for the job. We'll play a ball game just like the kind you're used to!"

A follow-up call revealed that getting to take part in the familiar activity of combination kickball had indeed helped to improve Ada's disposition. Meanwhile, my students enjoyed sending their greetings and hearing about the fitness program at Ada's new nursing home.

Glad Tidings

It is not unusual for a nursing home resident to return to the care of his family. He may, in fact, be looking forward to many happy and vigorous years during which he will live to a great extent autonomously.

When one of your fitness students leaves your fold with these bright prospects, talk with him about the importance of continuing his fitness program at home. Discuss how regular mental and physical exercise can help to keep him fit and able. If you have spare equipment such as an extra Nerf ball, then send him home with a tangible reminder to exercise.

When possible — and especially when the family is to play an important role in his care — meet with your student's family. Show them the equipment you use and tell them where to purchase or how to order it. Suggest books and video tapes that will help them to administer his at-home fitness program. Teach them games and exercises — enough to enable them to carry on his program without interruption when he leaves the facility.

When Students Get Ill

When a fitness student misses meetings due to illness, you should find out if the decline in his health is predicted to be temporary or permanent. If he has been taken to the hospital, make a note to visit him upon his return to the home. Drop by often to let the recuperating student know that you

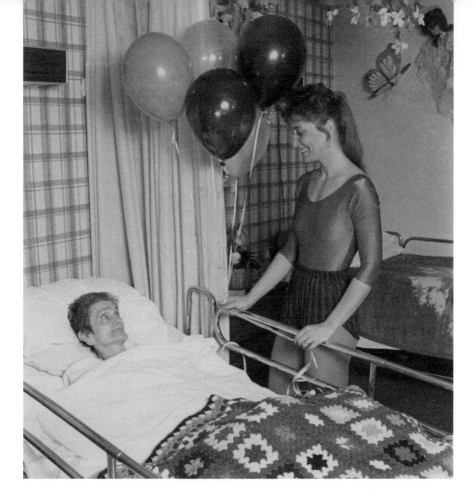

miss him in class and that the members look forward to his return.

When recovery is expected to take time (or when it is unknown if the student will ever be able to attend class again) look into the possibility of adding him to your one-on-one case load. Whether or not he is officially assigned to you as an individual student, remember that stopping by to say hello only takes a minute and can mean a lot to the person for whom extended bed rest has been prescribed.

Final Good-byes

Finally and inevitably, as a nursing home fitness leader you will be faced with learning to deal with the deaths of elderly students who have grown precious to you. When it happens you may wonder, What good is my fitness program if my members die? I hope that Luke's story will help to resolve the natural feelings of conflict and despair you can expect to experience when the time comes to grapple with this issue.

We started Luke's story back in Chapter Seven. When I first met Luke, a stroke survivor with serious emotional problems, he seemed irretrievably withdrawn and hopelessly disheartened. I remember thinking he was the saddest person that I had ever seen. It was an agreeable surprise, then, when he responded to plant therapy and subsequently accepted a program of strength and flexibility exercises.

But, as you have guessed, Luke died. When I heard the news I felt a heavy crush of impotence and remorse. Pessimistically, I dawdled alone in his room, plagued by self-doubts. Had I held out an implied promise of fitness to Luke? A promise as empty as his wheelchair in front of me?

As I pondered the relationship that had developed with this student a mental image of the man entered into my mind — not an image of Luke as he had been when I met him, with head lowered and dull blank eyes staring off into space, but an image of Luke as he was towards the end of his life. I saw him perk up as I entered the door, sit up proudly with a wide grin on his face, and hurl himself into a series of enthusiastic biceps curls before I even had time to say how-do-you-do. With this clear picture impressed on my mind, I knew that it had all been worth it. Right up to the end of his life Luke was mobile. And what's more, he was challenged. During his last months, instead of languishing in depression, Luke had known the satisfactions of achievement and success.

To summarize, it seems the rule that when circumstances are difficult for a person (and this applies to a person of any age) even the briefest moment of joy or the smallest award of positive feedback can lead to a disproportionate improvement in his attitude towards living. So, imagine the difference you can make by helping a person to secure these boons in substantial amounts and on a regular basis. Physical advances can be made. Psychological advances can be made. Greater mastery over the world around can be achieved. Self-sufficiency can be increased. Remember that by focusing on the positive you can open the door to blessings for yourself and for your elderly fitness students alike.

More Parting Thoughts

Our society is new at dealing with old age as we know it today. With vaccines and other technological breakthroughs, people are living longer lives. We have not yet discovered everything that can be accomplished in the quest to enjoy life to its fullest for the longest. In that sense, a revolution in modern thought is needed to turn our can't-do approach to aging into one of exploration and confident resolution.

Some daring prototypes of future lifestyle options are already being refined. Perhaps, for example, a practical goal for the geriatric fitness leader of the twenty-first century will be to help equip students to manage in congregate living centers, semi-protected environments in which the

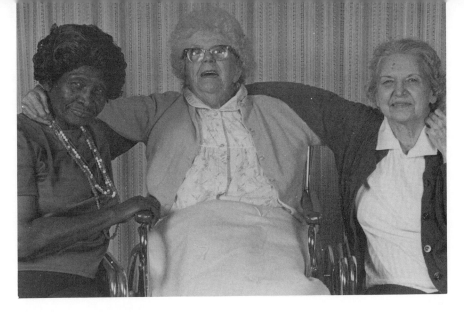

individual retains maximum independence.

At any rate, the post-war baby boomers, representing a massive population bulge, are growing older and, in the process, forcing society to look for ways to triumph over outdated concepts regarding the aging process. Accordingly, we are certain to see and hear more and more success stories as the years go by. And more than ever, we will need optimistic, spirited persons to render the services that our geriatric population requires.

And a Closing Word

Whether you work with a roomful of elderly fitness students or one-on-one with an individual family member, you belong to a unique group of pioneers in the field of geriatric care. You need never feel isolated or alone in your work, for there are many other devoted individuals striving to promote meaningful fitness activities for the oldest members of our society.

I know about these people firsthand thanks to the thrilling and unexpected reception that Seniorcise has been afforded both at the community level and at regional and national levels. As a result of media coverage and magazine articles about the program, I've had the pleasure of hearing from interested persons both near and far away. Some are professionals, some are volunteers, and some are lay persons with aging relatives. They form a diverse group, but they all have one thing in common: they care about the elderly. I hope that my book will prove useful to these hardworking and deserving people.

And I hope that you will enjoy boundless success in all of your geriatric fitness endeavors.

RECOMMENDED READING

Biegel, Leonard. (1984) *Physical Fitness and the Older Person: A Guide to Exercise for Health Care Professionals.* Rockville, Md.: Aspen Systems Corporation.

Coombs, Jan. (1984) *Living with the Disabled: You Can Help.* New York: Sterling Publishing Co., Inc.

Curtin, Sharon R. (1972) *Nobody Ever Died of Old Age.* Boston: Atlantic-Little, Brown and Company.

Fowler, Roy S. and W.E. Fordyce. (1974) *Stroke: Why Do They Behave That Way?* Dallas, Tx.: American Heart Association.

Hastings, Linda Emerson. (1981) *Complete Handbook of Activities and Recreational Programs for Nursing Homes.* Englewood Cliffs, N.J.: Prentice-Hall, Inc.

Krause, Richard. (1973) *Therapeutic Recreation Service: Principles and Practice* (3rd ed.). Philadelphia: Saunders College Publishing.

Lewis, Carole B. and Everett L. Smith (Eds.). (1985, October) *Topics in Geriatric Rehabilitation: Exercise and Aging,* Vol. 1, No. 1. Rockville, Md.: Aspen Systems Corporation.

Merrill, Toni. (1974) *Discussion Topics for Oldsters in Nursing Homes: 365 Things to Talk About.* Springfield, Il.: Charles C. Thomas.

Rosenberg, Magda. (1977) *Sixty-Plus & Fit Again.* New York: M. Evans and Company, Inc.

Ross, Mary Alice. (1984) *Fitness for the Aging Adult with Visual Impairment: An Exercise and Resource Manual.* New York: American Foundation for the Blind.

Sullivan, Margaret. (1987, July) Atrophy and Exercise. *Journal of Gerontological Nursing,* Vol. 13, No. 7. Thorofare, N.J.: SLACK, Inc., 26-31.

Thompson, Clem W. (1969) *Manual of Structural Kinesiology* (6th ed.). St. Louis, Mo.: The C.V. Mosby Company.

INDEX